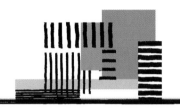

POSITIVE PSYCHIATRY

A Casebook

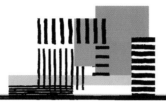

POSITIVE PSYCHIATRY

A Casebook

Edited by

Richard F. Summers, M.D.

Dilip V. Jeste, M.D.

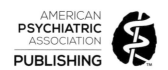

AMERICAN
PSYCHIATRIC
ASSOCIATION
PUBLISHING

If you wish to buy 50 or more copies of the same title, please go to www.appi.org/specialdiscounts for more information.

Copyright © 2019 American Psychiatric Association Publishing

ALL RIGHTS RESERVED

First Edition

Manufactured in the United States of America on acid-free paper
22   21   20   19   18   5   4   3   2   1

American Psychiatric Association Publishing
800 Maine Ave., S.W.
Suite 900
Washington, DC 20024-2812
www.appi.org

Library of Congress Cataloging-in-Publication Data
Names: Summers, Richard F., editor. | Jeste, Dilip V., editor. | American
    Psychiatric Association Publishing.
Title: Positive psychiatry : a casebook / edited by Richard F. Summers, Dilip V. Jeste.
Other titles: Positive psychiatry (2019)
Description: Washington, D.C. : American Psychiatric Association Publishing,
    [2019] | Includes bibliographical references and index.
Identifiers: LCCN 2018023614 (print) | LCCN 2018025265 (ebook) | ISBN
    9781615372010 (ebook) | ISBN 9781615371396 (pbk. : alk. paper)
Subjects: | MESH: Psychotherapy—methods | Happiness | Resilience, Psychological |
    Psychiatry—methods | Mental Disorders—therapy | Case Reports
Classification: LCC RC480.5 (ebook) | LCC RC480.5 (print) | NLM WM 40 | DDC
    616.89/14—dc23
LC record available at https://lccn.loc.gov/2018023614

British Library Cataloguing in Publication Data
A CIP record is available from the British Library.

For
Ronnie, Sam, and Claire
and
Kiran, Nischal, Neelum, Shafali, and Sonali

Contents

PART I

Mental Health Care

Section Editors:
Richard F. Summers, M.D., and Dilip V. Jeste, M.D.

PART III
Education and Coaching
Section Editor: Behdad Bozorgnia, M.D., M.A.P.P.

CONTRIBUTORS

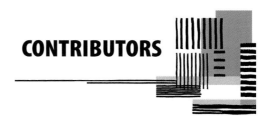

Keri Biscoe, M.D.
Ophthalmologist in Private Practice; Owner, St. Croix Eye Institute, LLC, Christiansted, St. Croix, U.S. Virgin Islands

Daniel S. Bowling III, J.D., M.A.P.P.
Senior Lecturing Fellow, Duke Law School, Durham, North Carolina; Assistant Instructor, Master of Applied Positive Psychology Program, University of Pennsylvania, Philadelphia, Pennsylvania

Behdad Bozorgnia, M.D., M.A.P.P.
Chief Resident of Outpatient Psychiatry, Department of Psychiatry, Hospital of the University of Pennsylvania, Philadelphia, Pennsylvania

Kathryn H. Britton, M.A.P.P.
Executive Coach, Theano Coaching and Silicon Valley Change Executive Coaching, Chapel Hill, North Carolina

Pollyanna V. Casmar, Ph.D.
Staff Psychologist, Department of Veterans Affairs, San Diego; Health Sciences Associate Professor, Department of Psychiatry, University of California, San Diego, La Jolla, California

Deanna C. Chaukos, M.D., F.R.C.P.C.
Assistant Professor, Division of Consultation Liaison Psychiatry, Department of Psychiatry, University of Toronto Faculty of Medicine; Psychiatrist, Mount Sinai Hospital, Joseph and Wolf Lebovic Health Complex, Toronto, Ontario, Canada

Ambrish S. Dharmadhikari, D.P.M., D.N.B., M.A.P.A.
Consultant Psychiatrist, Dr. H.D. Gandhi Memorial Hospital, Mumbai, Maharashtra, India

Joana Abed Elahad, M.S.
Medical Student, Rosalind Franklin University of Medicine and Science, Chicago, Illinois

Dilip V. Jeste, M.D.
Senior Associate Dean for Healthy Aging and Senior Care; Estelle and Edgar
Levi Chair in Aging; Distinguished Professor of Psychiatry and Neurosciences;
and Director, Sam and Rose Stein Institute for Research on Aging, University of California, La Jolla, California

Yash B. Joshi, M.D., Ph.D.
Third-Year Psychiatry Resident, Department of Psychiatry, University of California, San Diego, La Jolla, California

Kelsey T. Laird, Ph.D.
Postdoctoral Research Scholar, Semel Institute for Neuroscience and Human
Behavior, David Geffen School of Medicine at UCLA, Los Angeles, California

Helen Lavretsky, M.D., M.S.
Professor of Psychiatry In-Residence; Director, Late-Life Mood, Stress, and
Wellness Research Program, Semel Institute for Neuroscience and Human
Behavior, David Geffen School of Medicine at UCLA, Los Angeles, California

Ellen E. Lee, M.D.
Postdoctoral Research Fellow, Stein Institute for Research on Aging and Department of Psychiatry, University of California, La Jolla, California

Dan Li, B.A.
Medical Student, David Geffen School of Medicine at UCLA, Los Angeles,
California

Averria Sirkin Martin, Ph.D., L.M.F.T.
Staff Director of Research, Stein Institute for Research on Aging, University
of California, San Diego, La Jolla, California

Margot Montgomery O'Donnell, M.D.
Psychiatrist in Private Practice; Clinical Associate, Department of Psychiatry, Perelman School of Medicine, University of Pennsylvania, Philadelphia,
Pennsylvania

Marcela Ot'alora G., M.A., L.P.C.
Principal Investigator, Multidisciplinary Association for Psychedelic Studies, MDMA-Assisted Psychotherapy for PTSD, Boulder, Colorado

Andrew D. Penn, M.S., R.N., P.M.H.N.P.-B.C.
Associate Clinical Professor, University of California, San Francisco School of
Nursing; Psychiatric Nurse Practitioner, The Permanente Medical Group–
Redwood City, Redwood City, California

Shannon M. Polly, M.A.P.P., PCC
Leadership Coach and Executive Coach, Shannon Polly & Associates, Washington, D.C.

Charles L. Raison, M.D.
Mary Sue and Mike Shannon Chair for Healthy Minds, Children and Families; Professor, Human Development and Family Studies, School of Human Ecology; Professor, Department of Psychiatry, School of Medicine and Public Health, University of Wisconsin–Madison, Madison, Wisconsin

David C. Rettew, M.D.
Associate Professor of Psychiatry and Pediatrics; Director, Child and Adolescent Psychiatry Fellowship; Director, Pediatric Psychiatry Clinic, University of Vermont Larner College of Medicine, Burlington, Vermont

J. Greg Serpa, Ph.D.
Clinical Psychologist, VA Greater Los Angeles Healthcare System; Clinical Professor, UCLA Department of Psychology, West Los Angeles VA Medical Center, Los Angeles, California

Daniel D. Sewell, M.D.
Professor of Clinical Psychiatry; Co-director, Division of Geriatric Psychiatry; Associate Vice Chair, Department of Psychiatry, University of California, San Diego, La Jolla, California

Richard F. Summers, M.D.
Clinical Professor of Psychiatry and Senior Residency Advisor, Department of Psychiatry, Perelman School of Medicine, University of Pennsylvania, Philadelphia, Pennsylvania

Aviva Teitelbaum, M.D.
Clinical Assistant Professor of Psychiatry, SUNY Downstate Medical Center; Attending Psychiatrist, Opioid Treatment Program and Psychiatric Emergency Room, Kings County Hospital, Brooklyn, New York

Vihang N. Vahia, M.D., I.D.F.A.P.A.
Professor Emeritus, Department of Psychiatry, HBT Medical College and Dr. R.N. Cooper Municipal General Hospital; Consultant Psychiatrist, Breach Candy Hospital; Consultant Psychiatrist, Lilavati Hospital and Research Centre; Consultant Psychiatrist, Dr. H.D. Gandhi Memorial Hospital, Mumbai, Maharashtra, India

Disclosures of Competing Interests

The following contributors to this book have indicated a financial interest in or other affiliation with a commercial supporter, a manufacturer of a commercial product, a provider of a commercial service, a nongovernmental organization, and/or a government agency, as listed below:

Helen Lavretsky, M.D., M.S.—*Grant support:* Allergan, Alzheimer's Research and Prevention Foundation; National Center for Complementary and Integrative Health; National Institutes of Health/National Institute of Mental Health; Patient-Centered Outcomes Research Institute

David C. Rettew, M.D.—*Royalties: Psychology Today*

Daniel D. Sewell, M.D.—*Financial support:* Medical advisory board, Activ-Care Living–Residential Memory Care Inc.; *Research support:* Clinician participant, IDEAS Study; DHHS/HRSA Geriatric Workforce Enhancement Program Awards (The San Diego GWEP Collaborative; San Diego/Imperial Geriatric Education Center)

Richard F. Summers, M.D.—*Royalties:* Guilford Press

The following contributors to this book have indicated that they have no financial interests or other affiliations that represent or could appear to represent a competing interest with their contributions to this book:

Keri Biscoe, M.D.
Daniel S. Bowling III, J.D., M.A.P.P.
Behdad Bozorgnia, M.D., M.A.P.P.
Kathryn H. Britton, M.A.P.P.
Pollyanna V. Casmar, Ph.D.
Deanna C. Chaukos, M.D., F.R.C.P.C.
Ambrish S. Dharmadhikari, D.P.M., D.N.B., M.A.P.A.
Dilip V. Jeste, M.D.
Kelsey T. Laird, Ph.D.
Ellen E. Lee, M.D.
Dan Li, B.A.
Averria Sirkin Martin, Ph.D., L.M.F.T.
Margot Montgomery O'Donnell, M.D.
Marcela Ot'alora G., M.A., L.P.C.
Andrew D. Penn, M.S., R.N., P.M.H.N.P.-B.C.
Shannon M. Polly, M.A.P.P., PCC
J. Greg Serpa, Ph.D.
Aviva Teitelbaum, M.D.
Vihang N. Vahia, M.D., I.D.F.A.P.A.

FOREWORD

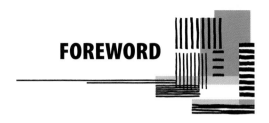

POSITIVE psychiatry, while less familiar to clinicians than positive psychology, expands the perspective of traditional clinicians. Rather than focusing exclusively on psychopathology, positive psychiatry includes the positive aspects of human life, including healthy strengths, traits, and communities. Positive psychiatry imagines a future where positive interventions not only reduce psychopathology but also enhance clinical medicine, positive emotions, and organizational management.

When I began to review this book, I was disappointed. The previous books that I had read on the practice of positive psychology were written by one or two authors. In contrast, the chapters that I read in this casebook were by many different authors whom I had not read before. As I explored further, I realized that this was genius. Positive psychiatry is an *art*, not just a technique. Being exposed to cases treated by a variety of *artists* deepened my understanding of the techniques of positive psychology in ways that were fresh and rewarding.

Particularly revealing, each chapter focuses on different psychiatric or medical disorders that earlier books on positive psychology do not address. Each chapter illustrates specific interventions that clinicians can adopt for their own practice. Resilience enhancement, strength-based interventions, and even positive emphasis to produce a remarkable remission in a case of chronic schizophrenia are illustrated. The use of MDMA as an adjunct in the psychotherapy of a woman struggling with severe posttraumatic stress disorder; mindfulness and meditation for caregivers of ill family members; and the use of positive principles in education and coaching round out the collection.

If the future imagined by positive psychology is to become a reality, we need these detailed case discussions by clinicians struggling with the complexities of real patients in the real world. This work takes its place among a number of important contemporary contributions in the area.

It is a particular pleasure for me to see the flourishing of positive psychiatry, as I am a psychiatrist and an early proponent of positive psychology. In order to *show* rather than *tell* about the novelty and power of positive psychiatry, I invite the readers of *Positive Psychiatry: A Casebook* to attend an open meeting of Alcoholics Anonymous (AA). This is one version of positive psychiatry lived and experienced. At an AA meeting, they will witness how a focus on positive emotions (the heart of positive psychology and psychiatry) can help heal an illness that kills 100,000 victims a year in the United States.

AA succeeds where medical treatment methods fail precisely because AA., like positive psychiatry, involves the positive rather than negative emotions. Positive emotion arises in the nonverbal subcortical limbic system, whereas conventional psychiatry values cognition, which arises in the cerebral cortex and upon words. There are three important emotions that AA and positive psychiatry use to affect the subcortical brain of the beginner: love, gratitude, and joy. The first three steps of AA keep it simple and can be distilled as "God is Love." Consider how the second and third steps open us to love by inviting us to believe "that a Power greater than ourselves could restore us to sanity" and to "make a decision to turn our lives over to God as we [understand] Him" along with the loving invitation to "[k]eep on coming back" to one's home group (the effective ingredient of AA).

Consider how the twelfth step embodies the heartfelt knowledge that to keep it, you have to give it away. This leads to the positive emotion of *joy*. Both principles are counterintuitive and militate against the world of cognitive enlightenment that has taken over modern rational psychiatry since the eighteenth century.

Long-term studies teach us that if the follow-up lasts longer than 2 years, moderation management, medication-assisted approaches (acamprosate, naltrexone), cognitive-behavioral therapy, and 28-day detoxification programs all usually fail to produce long-term abstinence. However, the only outcome that makes a lasting difference in the devastating disease called alcoholism—much as with nicotine dependence—is years of attending AA "home group"—sharing one's strength, hope, and experience with other alcoholics. This is how AA eventually succeeds in effecting stable abstinence

The AA mantras of "maintain an attitude of gratitude"—a major positive emotion—and "fake it 'til you make it" sound like utter hokum to my psychoanalytically trained ears. Then I reflect on my own 60-year prospective study of alcoholics, which revealed that 2,500 hours of long-term psychotherapy to 50 alcoholics produced only a single case of lifelong abstinence. In contrast, sticking with AA for 30 or more meetings, with its attitude of gratitude, eventually produced sustained abstinence in more than 80%!

The subcortical limbic system has no words, only heartfelt feelings. The importance of the limbic system to addiction has only been appreciated in the twentieth-first century with the advent of brain imaging (e.g., Nora Volkow) and research on the positive emotions (e.g., Julian Thayer, Antonio Damasio, Barbara Fredrickson). Thankfully, a half century before brain imaging, Bill W. devised a program that focused on the positive emotions.

AA succeeds because it catalyzes the reinforcement circuitry of limbic brain, hijacked by alcohol, to return to the purposes for which it was designed—to become attached to others. AA lovingly suggests that "the God of my understanding" can be reached by cultivating the positive emotions of faith, hope, love, joy, awe, forgiveness, compassion, and gratitude. Unbelievably, these emotions go unmentioned in most textbooks of psychology and psychiatry.

Over time, putting yourself in the loving embrace of a welcoming AA home group, replacing resentments with forgiveness and gratitude, and relishing the laughter of the AA group have much the same effect. Think of hugging puppies.

Unfortunately, the disease of alcoholism makes it very difficult for anybody but a fellow suffering, but now recovering, alcoholic to love or hug the alcoholic individual seeking help. For arrogant, resentful, narcissistic, bad-smelling drunks to step into a room where everybody once smelled like them, was as arrogant as them, and was even more resentful can be pure magic. Suddenly, they are loved, not because their priest or their Salvation Army worker feels sorry for them, but because they are *needed.* They are loved because they have arrived just in time to keep their future sponsors sober and in so doing save their lives. Saving lives produces joy.

Positive emotions, like joy, were not discussed academically until the twentieth century, until the advent of Martin Seligman and Barbara Fredrickson, but finally have emerged as an important new field of study and intervention. *Positive Psychiatry: A Casebook* advances this wonderful tradition by diving deeply into the particulars of individual histories and treatments and I expect it will help to influence psychiatry to become a more positive psychiatry.

George E. Vaillant, M.D.
Professor of Psychiatry, Harvard Medical School,
Boston, Massachusetts

Suggested Reading

Vaillant GE: Natural History of Alcoholism Revisited. Cambridge, MA, Harvard University Press, 1995

Vaillant GE: Positive Emotions and the Success of Alcoholics Anonymous. Alcoholic Treatment Quarterly 32:214–224, 2014

PREFACE

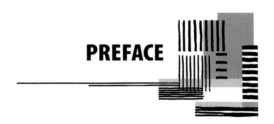

IF "the devil is in the details," then so are the angels. We began this casebook with curiosity about how clinicians and practitioners are using positive interventions in real clinical situations with real patients. General discussion of principles, theory, and techniques is extremely valuable, but we wanted to look more deeply into the details of actual treatments that employ these new approaches. *Positive Psychiatry: A Clinical Handbook*, edited by Jeste and Palmer and published in 2015, has been widely read and reviewed; and *Positive Psychiatry: A Casebook* takes another step in advancing the field. Positive interventions are compelling and interesting, and there is a growing empirical database, but as psychiatrists we wonder how we should be applying these ideas with our patients.

Positive psychiatry is a new field, with a developing literature and now a positive psychiatry caucus at the American Psychiatric Association as well as a positive psychiatry section at the World Psychiatric Association. Many practitioners have been inspired by positive psychology and are looking to apply these ideas in psychiatry and in medicine. The field is growing rapidly and has the potential to improve outcomes and change care systems.

Our goal is to illustrate how clinicians use traditional psychiatry approaches and positive interventions for particular patients, how positive interventions can enhance the quality of medical care, and how these interventions are employed in educational and coaching settings. The cases in this book are extensive and detailed, providing an opportunity for the reader to engage deeply in the clinical descriptions, decision making, and assessment of outcomes. Immersion in the cases will allow the reader to reflect on his or her practice and consider introducing these ideas and techniques as appropriate.

The book starts with an introduction to positive psychiatry. We provide an overview of the positive in the history of psychiatry, a summary of the effectiveness of positive interventions, and an overarching conceptualization of the field of positive psychiatry. Next are 13 chapters that present case studies. Each of the clinical and educational chapters includes a detailed history, the background of the person(s) seeking help, and a description of the interventions, framed by an assessment of each individual's strengths and vulnerabilities.

The 13 chapters are grouped into parts, representing these areas: mental health care, medical care, and education and coaching. The third part, illustrating positive interventions in nonclinical settings, provides a contrast with the clinical cases, allowing the reader a unique perspective on positivity. To our knowledge, this is the first compendium of psychiatric or positive case material to include such a wide array of settings.

We thank the contributing authors who graciously opened their professional lives and work to allow us to learn from their experiences. The authors articulate their understanding of their patients and how they chose the interventions offered. They reflect on their work and the outcome and effectiveness of the interventions.

We are deeply appreciative of the patients who agreed to allow their personal experiences and treatments to be written about. Of course, the information has been disguised to protect the privacy of the individuals. We recognize they have made an important contribution to advancing the field of positive psychiatry, and we are tremendously appreciative of their generosity.

Our thanks go to our many colleagues who have inspired and supported our interest in and commitment to positive psychiatry: Marty Seligman, Dan Blazer, George Vaillant, Robert Cloninger, James Pawelski, and Anthony Rostain. We thank Behdad Bozorgnia and Ellen Lee for their ideas and editorial work and Cassie Sacco for her administrative support. We are indebted to American Psychiatric Association Publishing, and particularly Bob Hales, Laura Roberts, and John McDuffie, for publishing the first positive psychiatry volume and for their outstanding editorial support for this work. Finally, we thank our wonderful wives and families for their love, support, and positivity!

Richard F. Summers, M.D.
Dilip V. Jeste, M.D.

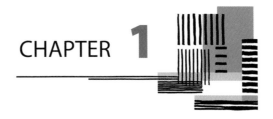

CHAPTER **1**

Overview of Positive Psychiatry

Behdad Bozorgnia, M.D., M.A.P.P.
Richard F. Summers, M.D.
Dilip V. Jeste, M.D.

WHAT IS POSITIVE PSYCHIATRY?

Psychiatry is typically defined as a branch of medicine focused on the study and treatment of mental illnesses. Accordingly, the field has aimed to reduce the symptoms caused by mental and behavioral disorders. This approach has led to important advances in the characterization and treatment of psychopathology; however, in that process, psychiatry has overlooked broader aspects of well-being among individuals with psychiatric disorders.

    Positive psychiatry may be defined as the science and practice of psychiatry that seeks to understand and promote well-being through assessments and interventions aimed at enhancing positive psychosocial factors among people who have or are at high risk for developing mental and physical illnesses (Jeste et al. 2015). It is an approach to mental health that seeks to expand the scope of psychiatry to the promotion of well-being in the overall population. Positive psychosocial factors include resilience, optimism, social engagement, wisdom, posttraumatic growth, hope, compassion, self-efficacy, and personal mastery, among others. As a branch of medicine, positive psychiatry is also focused on discerning the biological substrates of these traits, including their neurocircuitry, neurochemistry, and genetic basis, as well as developing biomarkers of these positive factors (Jeste et al. 2017). Importantly, positive psychiatry is intended not to replace traditional psychiatry but rather to complement it by shifting the focus from treating pathology to maintaining health and from treating symptoms to enhancing well-being.

As described below, positive psychology has been around for a long time. Thanks to the pioneering efforts of Martin Seligman and colleagues, the positive psychology movement has become popular even among the lay public. Remarkably, the movement has had little impact on practice, research, or training in psychiatry. Articles or book chapters on positive concepts in psychiatric journals or textbooks have been conspicuous by their absence. In 2012, when one of us (DVJ) googled the term *positive psychiatry*, he did not find a single published reference, although *positive psychology* had thousands of mentions in scientific and popular press. Positive psychiatry was DVJ's presidential theme during his tenure as president of the American Psychiatric Association in 2012–2013. The first book on positive psychiatry was published 2 years later (Jeste and Palmer 2015).

A BRIEF HISTORY OF POSITIVE PSYCHOLOGY

Auguste Rodin (1840–1917), a French sculptor who is considered the progenitor of modern sculpture, said, "I invent nothing. I just rediscover." It is a truism that there are no real inventions in this world. Almost all are only discoveries—they always existed in the past and will continue into the future. People merely reconceptualize age-old ideas into models that suit the time and place. Resilience, optimism, compassion, and wisdom have been described and discussed since the beginning of recorded human history. The value of these positive traits has long been emphasized in religious scriptures such as the Bible and the Indian Bhagavad Gita and in the writings of ancient Greek philosophers such as Aristotle and Plato, among others.

Positive psychology is a new field composed of old elements, and it is analogous to a musical remix that borrows parts from multiple sources to create an original whole. It interrogates ancient concepts with modern methodologies within a contemporary multicultural framework.

The idea of the positive has much older roots within the history of psychology. A thorough and exacting account of the history of positive psychology is well beyond the purposes of this chapter and is available to the curious reader elsewhere (see Linley et al. 2006).

Indeed, it may be argued that the study of the positive aspect of human experiences precedes the field of psychology itself considering that many of the ancient subjects, such as philosophy, literature, and religion, often entail rigorous and detailed explorations of the nature of "the good life." Two examples within the Western philosophical tradition are Plato's *Republic* and Aristotle's *Nicomachean Ethics*. In the *Republic*, Socrates engages his student Glaucon extensively on "the Form of the Good," which gives all other forms and thus knowledge their nature and meaning. Aristotle's classic work in the field of ethics contains an inquiry into the nature of the good that entails a theory of positive human traits, which he labels "virtues." Although the ideas of Plato and Aristotle are highly abstract and far removed from the practical world of human psychology, their focus on goodness and virtue as essential fields of inquiry highlights the historical depth of the positive within Western culture.

William James, a physician and psychologist, bears mentioning in the history of positive psychology. In his 1902 monograph, *The Varieties of Religious Experience*, he wrote about two categories of believers, namely "the healthy minded" and "the sick souled." He wrote, "In many persons, happiness is congenital and irreclaimable. 'Cosmic emotion' inevitably takes in them the form of enthusiasm and freedom. I speak not only of those who are animally happy. I mean those who, when unhappiness is offered or proposed to them, positively refuse to feel it, as if it were something mean and wrong" (James 1902/2017, p. 63).

The first use of the term *positive psychology* was by Abraham Maslow in his studies of "self-actualized" people during the 1950s. In *Toward a Psychology of Being*, Maslow (1962/2013) imagined a field that he labeled "'positive psychology,' or 'orthopsychology,' of the future in that it deals with fully functioning and healthy human beings, and not alone with normally sick ones." Maslow's core concepts and empirical research significantly contributed to humanistic psychology and paved the way for it to eventually become a large-scale systematic behavioral science.

Positive psychology uses empirical methodologies of social psychology to study "what makes life worth living." Therefore, positive psychology is distinct from "psychology as usual" in relation to what it investigates—namely, positive traits, positive states, positive institutions, and the ingredients that make up the good life. It intentionally moves away from the medical model adopted by clinical psychology and aims to identify and amplify the positive healthy states rather than address or ameliorate negative disease states. Thus, instead of studying phenomena such as depression and anxiety, positive psychologists study phenomena such as happiness and well-being.

A simple way to focus on the concept of the positive is to think of it as what people tend to want more of instead of less of. Therefore, positive psychology studies those parts of life that people value, and to some degree blurs the traditional fact-value distinction within the social sciences (Snyder et al. 2011). The positive is a culture-bound concept and will vary among different groups and traditions.

Martin Seligman introduced positive psychology as a distinct field of empirical psychology in the late 1990s. In his presidential address to the American Psychological Association, Seligman (1999) encouraged a shift in American psychology away from a field of science dedicated to the study of disease, distress, and overall negative or neutral phenomena, to "a reoriented science that emphasizes the understanding and building of the most positive qualities of an individual: optimism, courage, work ethic, future-mindedness, interpersonal skills, the capacity for pleasure and insight, and social responsibility" (Fowler et al. 1999, p. 559). In conceiving of positive psychology, Seligman and Csikszentmihalyi (2014) delineated two fundamental commitments of positive psychology: 1) to stray from the focus on suffering and instead focus on "positive subjective experience, positive individual traits, and positive institutions" and 2) to maintain positive psychology as a science that is subject to the same rigors and standards as any social science. With these two commitments they helped launch a field that has burgeoned over the past decades and is now well established within psychology with multiple peer-reviewed journals, national and international conferences, and several dedicated graduate programs in the United States and abroad.

THE POSITIVE IN THE HISTORY OF PSYCHIATRY

Although the concepts and practices of psychiatry have changed dramatically through the millennia, the central organizing subject matter has always remained mental illness. This understanding of psychiatry suggests that the field has little in common with—and, indeed, little to gain from—positive psychology, which proposes to investigate and amplify precisely that which is not diseased. Yet, a closer inspection of the history of psychiatry quickly reveals that the positive—that is, those elements of experience that define the good life—has always had a part within the world of psychiatry, though clearly not at center stage. The following strands of positive thought in psychiatry demonstrate that the positive had a place within the past of psychiatry and therefore will have a place within its future as well.

Sigmund Freud

Sigmund Freud, the father of psychoanalysis, is often quoted as emphasizing the importance of intrapsychic conflicts and the primacy of sexual and aggressive drives in explaining human behavior. He is hardly thought of as someone interested in the "positive" side of human life. In many works of positive psychology, Freud is mentioned as emblematic of the pessimistic and overly pathologizing attitude from which positive psychology is trying to distance itself (Sheldon and King 2001). Yet, a closer inspection of Freud's work quickly reveals that he did not exclusively investigate neurosis and character pathology, but also provided a rich theory investigating many positive human experiences and traits, such as wit, creativity, spirituality, sexuality, and love.

In his 1905 essay "The Joke and Its Relation to the Unconscious," Freud (1905/2003) provides an overview of jokes in terms of technique and structure before making a connection between the use of humor and his own psychoanalytic theory of the human mind. Indeed, "humor and playfulness" are listed as ubiquitously valued positive human traits in *Character Strengths and Virtues: A Handbook and Classification* by Chris Peterson and Martin Seligman (2004), which serves as positive psychology's nosological framework.

Freud's interest in the positive aspects of human nature extended further to include a very serious interest in the nature of human creativity. In such essays as "The Relation of the Poet to Day-Dreaming" (1908/1972), "The Theme of the Three Caskets" (1913/1958), and "The Moses of Michelangelo" (1914/1955), Freud establishes connections between the creative process of the artist and unconscious processes that result in neuroses, dreams, parapraxes, and so forth. His intent in these essays is to provide a theoretical explanation of human creativity as related to his broader theory of the human mind. Indeed, because of this contribution, Freud's work and its intellectual offspring are widely employed in contemporary understanding of art, literature, and film.

The fundamental goals and objectives of psychoanalysis and its purpose—that self-knowledge leads to freedom and greater agency—remind us that Freud's brainchild was based on the hope and belief that individuals could lead fuller, richer, and more satisfying lives. It was only as psychoanalysis sought greater connection with medicine that the emphasis on diagnosis and pathology became more pronounced.

Hans Loewald and the Vitality of the Unconscious

Throughout the middle to late twentieth century, the German-born psychoanalyst Hans Loewald made significant contributions to the world of psychiatry by synthesizing ego psychology and object relations theory and providing clarification on the mechanisms of change in psychoanalysis (see Chodorow 2003 for further discussion). Despite his contributions, he remains a somewhat underestimated figure in the world of psychoanalysis and an obscure figure in the world of psychology at large. Loewald took a developmental and process-oriented perspective on healing the human psyche, emphasizing that psychoanalysis allows for the resumption of normal development and that maturation is a perpetual process rather than a static achievement (Chodorow 2003). Loewald's contribution can be viewed as an example of the positive in psychiatry insofar as he framed psychopathology in terms of stunted healthy growth that can be rebooted by the attuned attention and interpretation of the analyst.

Loewald further emphasized the presence of the positive in the way he framed the unconscious and its relationship to experiences of vitality and psychological health. A common though misguided understanding of psychoanalytic literature emphasizes the unconscious as a kind of psychological underworld—teeming with irrational, incestuous, and destructive wishes, fantasies, and drives. Although Loewald does not discount the possibility of such "negative" aspects of the unconscious, he also shines light on the capacity of the unconscious to make human experience more vital and meaningful. He emphasizes the essential vitality of the unconscious in his discussion of transference phenomena: "Without such transference—of the intensity of the unconscious, of the infantile ways of experiencing life which has no language and little organization, but the indestructibility and power of the origins of life…without such transference, or to the extent to which such transference miscarries, human life becomes sterile and an empty shell" (Loewald 1960, p. 12). Far from viewing the unconscious as solely a source of disease and deficiency, Loewald emphasizes the positive aspects of the unconscious—those that lead to human creativity, authenticity, and a deep sense of meaning in life.

Erik Erikson and the Developmental Perspective

Since its inception by Freud, psychoanalytic theory has used a developmental model of the psyche to explain psychopathology. Erik Erikson extended the developmental model into adulthood and posited that the human life cycle consists of eight distinct stages centered around the resolution or persistence of archetypal conflicts pertinent to each particular stage (Erikson 1959).

The successful navigation and resolution of each stage involves the development of a strength or virtue. Thus, the course of a healthy human life entails the development of hope, will, purpose, competence, fidelity, love, care, and wisdom. At least three of these virtues (love, hope, wisdom) are mentioned verbatim in Peterson and Seligman's (2004) book on character strengths and virtues, whereas most others have close approximations in their book (e.g., will and courage, competence and self-regulation). Erikson's theory posits a developmental progression of positive traits and explicitly links these traits to the successful resolution of specific conflicts. His work lacks the rigorous empirical basis of modern positive psychology but stands out as a contribution to understanding positivity.

George Vaillant: Defenses and Mental Health

George Vaillant, in his book *The Wisdom of the Ego* (Vaillant 1993) and his writing about the Harvard Study of Adult Development (Vaillant 2008), provides an in-depth exploration of the positive side of mental defense mechanisms. He regards defense mechanisms as processes that are fundamental to mental health, adult development, and creativity. Vaillant catalogues a series of defense mechanisms, ranging from immature psychotic mechanisms (e.g., projection), to neurotic mid-level mechanisms (e.g., intellectualization), to mature defense mechanisms (e.g., altruism). The crucial difference between immature and mature defenses is the ability to synthesize conflicting feeling states and realities rather than merely denying them in simplistic or convoluted fashion.

Vaillant's innovation lies in his shift in emphasis from using the ideas of ego psychology solely to explain mental illness to using those ideas to create a positive notion of mental health. He posits that the "actions of the ego" or the defenses are the means by which human beings achieve mental health and are not merely the mechanism of disease. Furthermore, he demonstrates that the defense mechanisms used in achieving mental health are distinct entities that are not merely the absence of immature defense mechanisms.

Irvin Yalom and Salvation by Death

Irvin Yalom is well known for his contribution to both group and existential psychotherapies. His clinical work focused on the four main existential concerns: freedom, death, isolation, and meaninglessness (Yalom 1980). Yalom and others also frame these existential imperatives as living with authenticity, wisdom, and courage. Drawing from the works of Yalom as well as other existential psychotherapists and philosophers, Roger Bretherton explores the symbiotic relationship between existentialism and positive psychology and challenges the notion that existentialism is inherently pessimistic (Bretherton and Ørner 2004). He draws attention to the overlapping concern of both schools of thought with character strengths, and points out the potential ability for existentialism to add theoretical depth to the empirical data of positive psychology.

Beyond his contribution to existential psychology, Yalom's contribution to the field of thanatology, or the study of death, also has a positive dimension. Through both his books on psychotherapy and his novels, Yalom often points out that the thought of death brings an opportunity for psychological growth.

Supportive Psychotherapy: Out With the Bad, In With the Good

Traditionally, psychodynamic psychotherapy is conceived as a continuum with expressive therapy at one end and supportive therapy at the other end (Siqueland and Barber 2002). Expressive therapy is based on analyzing a person's natural psychological defenses and bringing unconscious conflicts into awareness. Open-ended questioning and allowing the patient to free-associate are often the means by which this is done. Supportive psychotherapy, on the other hand, is aimed at "supporting what is already there" rather than questioning a person's defense mechanisms and delving deeply into his or her unconscious mind. Supportive interventions attempt to increase a person's self-esteem, psychological functioning, and adaptive skills through a combination of reassurance, reframing, and guidance (Gabbard 2009).

The mechanism of supportive psychotherapy is defined as improved reality testing, enhanced self-esteem, a decrease in dysfunctional behaviors, and a corrective emotional experience facilitated by the therapeutic "holding environment." Summers and Lord, however, regard supportive psychotherapy as applied positive psychology and suggest a new mechanism by which it achieves its ends—namely, "new positive experiences—increased positive affect, increased engagement, and more effective utilization of strengths" (Summers and Lord 2015, p. 212). Their work suggests a deep confluence between supportive psychotherapy and positive psychology ideas and techniques.

Supportive therapy has complex and deep roots in the history of psychotherapy. Initially, psychoanalysts aimed to differentiate the work of psychoanalysis from other therapeutic techniques that worked through "suggestion." As early as the 1930s, however, analysts such as Edward Glover began to question why psychotherapy that is not entirely psychoanalytic was showing effective results. He suggested that such therapy worked because the "inexact interpretations" provided allowed patients to focus their minds away from their anxiety-provoking core conflict and thus bolster their already existing defenses (Rockland 2003). In 1951, Merton Gill suggested a style of therapy designed to "strengthen the ego." To this end, he suggested ways to "to encourage, praise, or in general, to give narcissistic support for those ego activities in which defense is combined with adaptive gratifications" (p. 66). This shift from defining and diminishing the psychopathology of the patient to elucidating and amplifying positive traits and states is consistent with positive psychology. Thus, the orientation of positive psychology in focusing on strengths and creating new positive experiences does not represent a complete break from the tradition of psychiatry and psychotherapy, but rather a new way of looking at the very old and well-established tradition of supportive psychotherapy.

Oral Tradition of Supervision

Beyond specific theorists and concepts, psychiatry has a long tradition of using clinical supervision as a means to educate and develop budding psychotherapists. In supervision, a more experienced psychotherapist mentors and teaches a less-experienced psychotherapist through the detailed discussion of a patient. Within this context, there has been a long tradition of focusing on the patient's strengths to foster healing and psychological growth in the context of psychotherapy. Informally, we have observed that many clinicians report that their most helpful supervision experiences have steered them toward a nuanced combination of disease amelioration and supportive enhancement of patients' strengths, and patients' ability to form a therapeutic alliance requires warmth, engagement, and positivity. We have found it interesting how infrequently these "pearls of wisdom" found their way into theory and publication until the formal development of the field of positive psychology.

The Recovery Movement

The recovery movement in psychiatry redefines the aims of treatment as centered on the consumer rather than the clinician (Resnick and Rosenheck 2006). This recent trend distinguishes clinical from personal recovery: *clinical recovery* emphasizes the traditional psychiatric imperatives of symptom relief, social functioning, relapse prevention, and risk management, and *personal recovery* emphasizes individual aims of personal strengths, authenticity, and meaning in life (Slade 2010). Many large community mental health systems are reorganizing services along consumer-focused lines and employing recovered individuals as part of the treatment team or as supports for patients in navigating care. This approach clearly reflects central ideas in positive psychology because the emphasis is on the patient's personal strengths, positive experiences, and visions of the good life in the service of patient well-being.

In conclusion, the positive has a long-standing place in the history of psychiatry. We hope to show through the cases in this book that many of these themes are reflected in the contemporary conceptualization of positive psychiatry and the application of these ideas in clinical and nonclinical settings.

A BRIEF SUMMARY OF POSITIVE INTERVENTIONS

After nearly 20 years of research, positive psychology has developed a considerable empirical understanding of happiness, resilience, positive relationships, positive emotions, and many other related topics. We focus in the remainder of this overview on those evidence-based interventions meant to increase happiness, subjective well-being, and overall flourishing, the so-called positive interventions.

Positive psychology interventions do seem to work. Bolier et al. (2013) pooled data from 39 studies of positive psychology interventions used in randomized controlled trials (RCTs). They found that positive psychology interventions show a small but statistically significant effect size on boosting subjective and psychological well-being. Similarly, they found that these interventions show a small but significant effect size for reducing symptoms of depression. In studies in which long-term (3-month to 1-year) follow-up data were available, positive psychology interventions showed a small but significant effect size for subjective and psychological well-being but no significant effect for depression. In a subgroup analysis, the authors found that effect sizes tend to increase with longer, individual, face-to-face interventions, and with interventions aimed at populations with specific psychosocial problems or populations referred from health care centers. Interestingly, because this review and casebook are about a combination of positive interventions in treatment settings, we may be able to access these more robust effects, albeit at individual or anecdotal level.

In the following subsections, we review a few of the interventions with the strongest evidence. Each subsection includes a brief background about the intervention and a summary of the findings from various relevant studies.

Positive Intervention: Gratitude

One of the most commonly used and researched positive psychology interventions to promote positive states is the *gratitude exercise*. Generally, gratitude interventions entail either writing a gratitude list or making a gratitude visit, which involves reading aloud a letter expressing gratitude to the person toward whom one feels grateful.

In their review, Wood et al. (2010) refer to two perspectives on gratitude: one that views gratitude as an emotion and the other that views gratitude as a broader character trait or life orientation. From the first perspective, gratitude is seen as a singular emotional response to a perceived benefit from some source outside of the self, most frequently another person. Gratitude, in this sense, is an interpersonal emotion that is largely focused on appreciating the positive actions of other people. For other researchers, however, this view is too narrow and does not capture the fundamental and broad nature of gratitude. These researchers define *gratitude* more in terms of a trait or life orientation. By analyzing the data regarding gratitude from a variety of gratitude scales, including the Gratitude Questionnaire—Six-Item Form (GQ-6; McCullough et al. 2002), the Appreciation Scale (Adler and Fagley 2005), and the Gratitude, Appreciation, and Resentment Test (GRAT; Watkins et al. 2003), these researchers, as discussed by Wood et al., concluded that gratitude has nine subdimensions. These components represent individual differences in the experience of grateful affect, appreciation of other people, a focus on what the person has, feelings of awe when encountering beauty, behaviors to express gratitude, a focus on the positive in the present moment, appreciation rising from understanding that life is short, a focus on the positive in the present moment, and positive social comparisons.

Although the results are not entirely consistent, about 12 RCTs have now demonstrated that gratitude can be increased and that doing so often results in decreased depression, decreased anxiety, decreased body dissatisfaction, improved sleep quality, increased happiness, increased well-being, and increased life satisfaction (Wood et al. 2010). Some methodological shortcomings may have skewed the results of these studies, including the common use of nonactive or nocebo (writing down hassles) control groups, small study samples, and the almost exclusive use of self-report scales to measure outcomes. Despite the need for further research, gratitude may serve as a relatively easy-to-use positive intervention that poses low risk and may confer meaningful benefit to patients, when used in proper and individually tailored fashion.

Gratitude has several correlates, including less psychopathology, greater well-being, more positive relationships, and perhaps even better health (Wood et al. 2010). In a large cross-sectional study, Kendler et al. (2003) showed that gratitude correlated with significantly diminished lifetime risk of major depressive disorder, generalized anxiety disorder, specific phobia, substance abuse, and bulimia nervosa. Kashdan et al. (2006) showed that in people with posttraumatic stress disorder, higher levels of gratitude correlated not only with diminished symptoms but also with significantly higher functioning. Multiple studies have shown that gratitude correlates with increased life satisfaction, lower negative affect, higher positive affect, and even increased eudaimonic well-being (Wood et al. 2010). In addition, gratitude correlates with both self- and peer-reported quality of relationships (Wood et al. 2010).

There is emerging evidence that gratitude is correlated with decreased overall stress, which could be related to improved health outcomes (Wood et al. 2009). Although the majority of these studies are cross-sectional and cannot determine causality, gratitude is an important component of mental health. There are also RCTs demonstrating that gratitude interventions lead to improved sleep quality through the mechanism of decreased negative sleep thoughts (Emmons and McCullough 2003; Wood et al. 2009).

Character Strengths and Virtues

In addition to promoting positive states such as gratitude, positive psychology has focused on the study and promotion of positive traits, also known as character strengths. Quinlan et al. (2012) discuss various systematic conceptions and ways to measure character strengths. The most thoroughly researched system is Character Strengths and Virtues (Peterson and Seligman 2004), a typology of 24 character strengths composed of specific constellations of thinking, feeling, and behaving. After performing a broad literature search of traits that were ubiquitously morally valued across cultures and that contribute to both personal and community betterment, Peterson and Seligman determined that the character strengths cluster around six organizing virtues: justice, humanity, courage, temperance, wisdom, and transcendence. Each of these virtues entails various character strengths that represent the specific manifestation of the virtue in human behavior. For example, curiosity is a manifestation of wisdom, whereas self-regulation is an incarnation of temperance. Unlike other valued human traits, such as talents, the character strengths and virtues represent moral traits that may manifest more naturally in some individuals but are subject to willful development in everyone (Peterson and Seligman 2004).

Peterson and Seligman (2004) also created the Values in Action (VIA) Survey of Character Strengths, a 240-item self-report questionnaire aimed at measuring the character strengths. The VIA has shown good reliability and validity, been translated into a wide variety of languages, and been subject to a variety of factor analyses. For individuals younger than 18 years, there is an equally valid and reliable version, the VIA Youth Survey (VIA-YS; Park and Peterson 2006).

In a global sample, the most common strengths were kindness, fairness, honesty, gratitude, and judgment, whereas the least common were prudence, modesty, and self-regulation (Park et al. 2006). The character strengths most commonly correlated with subjective well-being are zest, hope, curiosity, love, and gratitude. Those least correlated with subjective well-being are appreciation of beauty and excellence, creativity, kindness, and love of learning (Park et al. 2004).

Although the studies are somewhat heterogeneous in nature, there is emerging evidence that strength-based interventions have a small but consistent positive effect on subjective well-being (Quinlan et al. 2012). Strength-based interventions generally consist of identifying strengths using the VIA or another measure and then encouraging the participant to use the strength in a new way at a particular frequency. Some studies recommend that the participants use their top or signature strengths, others have suggested that participants use their least commonly used strengths, and still others have suggested the use of specific strengths (e.g., zest, hope, gratitude) (Mitchell et al. 2009; Proyer et al. 2013; Rust et al. 2009; Seligman et al. 2005). The studies have a wide variety of follow-up times, ranging from 2 months to 2 years. There is no consensus on the optimal intensity, duration, and frequency of interventions.

The most consistent finding across studies is that using strengths on a regular basis increases people's well-being, as measured in large part through the Life Satisfaction Survey. There is less of a consistent effect of using strengths on hedonic well-being as measured through the Positive and Negative Affect Schedule (PANAS) or on overall functioning as measured through academic achievement (Quinlan et al. 2012). Some studies have also shown a significant lowering of depressive symptoms (Seligman et al. 2005), but others have failed to replicate such results, in large part because the placebo groups in these studies have also shown a robust antidepressant response (Gander et al. 2013; Mongrain and Anselmo-Matthews 2012). As with gratitude exercises, many unanswered questions remain regarding use of character strengths; however, the evidence suggests that character strengths, like gratitude exercises, entail low likelihood of harm while representing a small but significant benefit on well-being as well as other positive outcomes such as academic achievement.

Optimism and Hope

A variety of interventions within the literature of positive psychology point to the importance of hope and optimism in fostering subjective well-being. In a large meta-analysis of over 300 studies, Alarcon et al. (2013) found that hope and optimism are related but distinct character traits that are unique when compared with other personality inventories. They showed that optimism is positively related to subjective well-being, life satisfaction, happiness, and physical health, and negatively related to depression and anxiety, and that hope is associated positively with happiness and negatively with depression and stress. The studies suggest that optimism and hope are related to overall psychological well-being because they act as psychological resources within themselves and predispose individuals to the acquisition of further resources. For example, a hopeful and optimistic individual may be happier because she sees the future as bright, and this outlook serves as a source of happiness in and of itself. Also, this belief leads to actions that result in the acquisition of further resources for happiness, such as making more friends and asking for a job promotion.

Although hope and optimism are distinct concepts, both entail positive expectations of the future, and there is a correlation between the two ($r=0.66$) (Gallagher and Lopez 2009). Within the positive psychology literature, the term *hope* generally refers specifically to the understanding of hope within C.R. Snyder's hope theory. Snyder (2002) conceives of hope as fundamentally a "positive motivational state," composed of three distinct cognitive components—goals, agency, and pathways—which refer to desired outcomes, adequate energy to achieve the goals, and the means of achieving the goals, respectively.

Optimism has a diverse yet coherent set of definitions ranging from those pertaining to expectancy to those pertaining to explanation. From the expectancy perspective, optimism entails a mind-set that believes good things will be plentiful in the future and bad things scarce. Other expectancy definitions of optimism refer to a tendency to expect positive outcomes or to look on the bright side of things. Optimism is thus temporal and entails a tendency to frame the future in a desirable light. From the perspective of expectancy, researchers commonly measure optimism or pessimism using the Life Orientation Test—Revised (LOT-R; Herzberg et al. 2006).

Martin Seligman's proposed view of optimism is based on cognitive explanatory style (Gillham et al. 2001). The specific pattern of thoughts that individuals use to explain events to themselves determines their particular explanatory style. Explanatory styles can be characterized along the dimensions of *permanence*, or relation to temporality; *pervasiveness*, or relation to locale/space; and *personalization*, or relation to external or internal sources.

An optimistic explanatory style entails thinking about negative events in ways that are temporary, are location specific, and allot control to the self. Consequently, optimists explain positive events in terms that are permanent, pervasive, and internal to the self. For example, if an optimist does well on a test, she thinks, "I did well because I am a hard worker." In response to a good grade, a pessimist might respond, "I did well because I got lucky." A pessimistic explanation places the cause of a good outcome outside the self in a way that is temporary and location bound (i.e., luck). From an explanatory style perspective, researchers use the Attributional Style Questionnaire (ASQ; Peterson et al. 1982) to measure relative optimism and pessimism. Compared with gratitude and character strengths, optimism and hope are not as thoroughly or rigorously explored.

Despite some theoretical ambiguity, multiple studies have shown that interventions aimed at increasing optimism and hope result in increased subjective well-being and decreased depressive symptoms (Cheavens et al. 2006; Gillham et al. 1995, 2007; Layous et al. 2013; Peters et al. 2010; Seligman 2007; Sheldon and Lyubomirsky 2006). Varying methods are used to boost optimism and hope. Some interventions simply encourage participants to be more optimistic. Others promote writing about optimism or hope at a particular frequency (generally once a day) for a particular duration (generally around 1 week). The specific writing instructions vary; examples include 1) having participants write down events that they are looking forward to in a detailed and vivid manner for 6 days in a row and 2) having participants imagine "their best future self" for 20 minutes at a time for 3 days in a row. Beyond these writing-based interventions, there are more elaborate and involved interventions that are meant to boost resilience by teaching the basics of cognitive-behavioral therapy (e.g., the cognitive model and the thought record) and encouraging participants to reframe their automatic thoughts toward a more optimistic explanatory style.

Somatic Positive Interventions

Almost all positive psychology interventions focus exclusively on the mind as a means to enhance human experience, although some research has entailed somatic interventions to enhance human functioning and experience. Positive somatic interventions use physiological and bodily means to achieve greater human well-being in a manner that preserves and promotes health in the long term. Such somatic interventions include positive psychonutraceuticals, physical activity, positive psychopharmacology, and sexuality.

POSITIVE PSYCHONUTRACEUTICALS

Food is rarely thought of within the academic psychological and psychiatric community as a means to enhance well-being. While there is emerging literature on the effects that various types of food and different eating behaviors can have on subjective well-being, the relationship between food and psyche is underexplored. Outside of science, however, the relationship between food and mental well-being is firmly established. As the American essayist Wendell Berry (1992) writes, "Eating with the fullest pleasure—pleasure, that is, that does not depend on ignorance—is perhaps the profoundest enactment of our connection with the world. In this pleasure we experience and celebrate our dependence and our gratitude, for we are living from mystery, from creatures we did not make and powers we cannot comprehend" (p. 326).

In a RCT, Macht and Dettmer (2006) demonstrated that consuming an apple or a bar of chocolate, compared with eating nothing, significantly enhanced mood up to 90 minutes postconsumption. Furthermore, of the three conditions, eating chocolate induced more joy in participants. Chocolate's effects, however, were not wholly positive, because participants also tended to experience more guilt after consuming chocolate than after eating an apple or nothing. It is important to avoid a simplistic pharmacological interpretation of the results, which claims that it is the chemical constituents of chocolate as opposed to the experience of eating chocolate that results in its psychological effects (Michener and Rozin 1994). The study suggests that the relationship between food and emotions is complex but an important area for further exploration as a positive intervention.

PHYSICAL ACTIVITY

A second example of a somatic positive intervention is physical activity. In a meta-analysis of more than 400 studies with about 13,000 participants, Reed and Ones (2006) found that aerobic exercise significantly increased positive affect for at least 30 minutes following the cessation of activity, with an overall moderate to large effect size. In a meta-analysis of over 39 RCTs with data from more than 2,000 participants, Cooney et al. (2014) found that physical exercise led to a small to moderate reduction in depressive symptoms. In another meta-analysis, Stubbs et al. (2017) examined data from six RCTs with 262 adult participants and found that, compared with active and passive control subjects, exercise demonstrated a significant and moderate effect on reducing anxiety symptoms.

A plethora of studies have found that physical activity leads to improved subjective well-being in both clinical and nonclinical populations (Crews et al. 2004; Heller et al. 2004; McLafferty et al. 2004). Many studies suggest that exercise correlates with subjective well-being; however, most of these studies were not randomized trials, and therefore no causal conclusion can be drawn. More research is needed to provide definitive answers regarding the effects of exercise on well-being in a positive sense.

POSITIVE PSYCHOPHARMACOLOGY

Positive psychopharmacology, or "cosmetic psychopharmacology," is a field that suggests the use of chemical means to enhance human experience and functioning (Rosenthal and Westreich 2010). Traditionally, psychopharmacology uses the medical model to tailor a particular treatment to a disease, but positive psychopharmacology suggests that chemicals can be used to enhance performance or happiness and not simply to treat disease. The idea is controversial, and very little consensus exists in the field of bioethics on the topic. The central conflict about positive psychopharmacology is between people who devalue the idea of using medicines for enhancement (pharmacological Calvinism) and people who support using pharmacology for all types of human ends outside of the treatment of disease (pharmacological utopianism) (Stein 2012a).

An example of positive psychopharmacology is the ingestion of a substance that some readers may be ingesting as they read this very sentence: caffeine. Some evidence suggests that through adenosine antagonism, intracellular calcium mobilization, and phosphodiesterase inhibition, caffeine improves cognitive performance while also increasing the perception of alertness and wakefulness. Importantly, there is ample evidence that caffeine also induces anxiety, thus demonstrating the potential harms of positive psychopharmacology and emphasizing the importance of judicious use of any substance for intended beneficial purposes (Cappelletti et al. 2015).

Stimulant medications have long been used by nonclinical populations as a means of cognitive enhancement. According to the National Survey on Drug Use and Health, 8.5% of the population age 12 years and older used stimulant medications for nonmedical purposes (Snodgrass and LeBaron 2008). In a systematic review of stimulant use for nonmedical purposes, Smith and Farah (2011) reviewed 28 articles and found that the majority of the evidence suggests that stimulant use improves declarative memory and that some evidence shows that stimulant use may enhance consolidation of memories. There is less evidence that stimulant use optimizes working memory and cognitive control. These authors conclude that more research is needed on the topic to provide a better picture of the neurocognitive effects of stimulants in healthy populations; however, such research is difficult due to a lack of funding sources (Smith and Farah 2011).

Nonmedical stimulant use is not without risk. Some evidence suggests that the earlier a person uses nonmedical stimulants, the greater his or her odds are for developing an addiction to prescription drugs (McCabe et al. 2007). Further, the U.S. Food and Drug Administration has placed a black box warning on stimulant medications for increased risk of sudden death in patients with preexisting cardiac disease, stroke, myocardial infarction, hypertension, and increased heart rate. Stimulants have benefits but also serious side effects that warrant not only further study but also carefully monitored use in any setting.

Throughout human history, various cultures have used hallucinogenic substances for a variety of practices, including inducing existentially and spiritually meaningful experiences. There is an emerging body of literature on the uses of hallucinogens for enhancing meaning and promoting subjective well-being in healthy adults. Griffiths et al. (2008) conducted a double-blind RCT in 36 healthy volunteers, comparing the effects of high-dose oral psilocybin with those of oral methylphenidate in a controlled study setting. They found that compared with the methylphenidate group, the psilocybin group had significantly higher retrospective ratings of positive attitudes, mood, social effects, and behavior at 2-month and 14-month follow-ups. Furthermore, at 14-month follow-up, 64% of the volunteers concluded that the psilocybin experience increased their sense of well-being or life satisfaction moderately or very much. These results were consistent with those from a 2006 study, in which volunteers, at 2-month follow-up, rated the psilocybin experience as having substantial personal meaning and spiritual significance, which led to positive changes in attitudes and behavior, as corroborated by community observers (Griffiths et al. 2006). In another RCT, Griffiths et al. (2016) showed that, compared with an active placebo, psilocybin led to decreases in depression, overall anxiety, and death anxiety, while also increasing quality of life, life meaning, and optimism. Studerus et al. (2011) found that in 110 healthy participants, psilocybin induced profound changes in mood, perception, thought, and self-experience in a dose-dependent fashion, with a majority of subjects describing the experience as pleasurable, enriching, and nonthreatening. Importantly, in a minority of the participants, psilocybin led to significant anxiety and distress, which were, however, managed with reassurance by the investigators. Further research is needed to replicate these findings in larger samples; however, currently psilocybin remains a promising form of positive psychopharmacology.

SEXUALITY

Another area of somatic positive interventions is sexuality, which, despite a number of promising results, remains a highly understudied area of human psychology and behavior. In a Swedish sample, Brody and Costa (2009) found that the frequency of penile-vaginal intercourse correlated with satisfaction with life. In an international sample of more than 25,000 participants, Laumann et al. (2006) found that sexual well-being independently correlated with happiness in general even when controlling for such factors as depression and physical health. There are many cross-sectional studies that suggest a strong relationship between sexual satisfaction and life satisfaction in general (Davison et al. 2009; Holmberg et al. 2010; Hooghe 2012). None of these studies are experimental, and thus they are subject to various confounding factors. Sexuality, however, remains a promising and underdeveloped area of research on human well-being.

Special Topics in Positive Psychiatry

Positive Child and Adolescent Psychiatry

The field of child and adolescent psychiatry, steeped in the developmental perspective of mental functioning, is a fertile ground for the principles of positive psychiatry to grow. Many child psychiatrists do incorporate most tenets of a positive psychiatry approach. Yet, child psychiatry has not escaped the predominant emphasis on a disease model focused on psychopathology, as illustrated by the recent dramatic increase in psychotropic medication use (Olfson et al. 2012). There is also strong evidence that most of the core domains of child psychopathology exist along broad spectrums, with few qualitative boundaries, among those with low, average, or high levels of a particular behavior (Rettew 2013).

Positive Psychiatry of Aging

Counteracting the prevalent ageist notions about aging being inevitably associated with progressive functional decline, numerous studies have reported on successful aging (Carstensen et al. 2003; Jeste et al. 2010, 2013). There is considerable evidence from neuroscience research that neuroplasticity, with brain growth and development, can continue into old age when there is adequate physical, cognitive, and psychosocial stimulation. This neuroplasticity likely enables positive psychological traits to affect individuals' health throughout the life span, although the brain is less plastic in later life than in youth.

Positive Psychiatry for Serious Mental Illnesses

The United Nations formally recognized pursuit of happiness as a fundamental human goal, but little attention has been given to the experience of happiness among people with serious mental illnesses such as schizophrenia. Currently, treatments for these illnesses typically are designed to target positive symptoms and prevent relapse. Persons with serious mental illnesses benefit most from concrete, skill-based strategies that are a component of positive psychological interventions. Meyer et al. (2012) conducted a pilot study of a group positive psychotherapy, called Positive Living, in 16 outpatients with schizophrenia. The intervention included elements designed to address common cognitive impairments associated with schizophrenia; elements included asking participants to report on an ongoing positive goal in each session, beginning and ending every session with a brief mindfulness exercise ("mindfulness minute"), and creating worksheets for each positive psychology exercise. Participants reported significant improvements in well-being, savoring, hope/confidence, goal orientation, and psychotic and other psychological symptoms postintervention and 3 months later. Using positive interventions in conjunction with traditional psychosocial treatments such as cognitive-behavioral therapy, social skills training, or psychoeducation may enhance an individual's progress toward recovery. Positive psychiatry for serious mental illness is not an oxymoron; rather, it is a much-needed approach to fully addressing the toll of these disorders in terms of suffering and reduced well-being. At the very least, positive psychiatry provides a more humanistic approach that avoids reductionism.

Positive Psychiatry and Medical Education

The level of physician burnout and depression has reached epidemic proportions across the United States. Among American medical students, rates of burnout are close to 50%, while rates of suicidality range from 10% to 12% (Dyrbye et al. 2008). For residents, burnout seems to reach as high as 76% in some studies (McCray et al. 2008). This has lead to an increasing amount of interest in physician wellness and resilience as a means to prevent burnout (Eckleberry-Hunt 2009). A recent meta-analysis by West et al. (2016) showed that positive interventions on a systemic and individuate level can both improve well-being and prevent burnout. Positive psychiatry is becoming increasingly important in medical education.

CONCLUSIONS AND FUTURE DIRECTIONS

The Jeste and Palmer (2015) book *Positive Psychiatry: A Clinical Handbook* launched the public discussion about the combination of psychiatry and positive psychology approaches. Summers and Lord (2015) created a conceptual framework for applying both positive and traditional psychotherapeutic techniques based on a patient's particular symptoms and strengths. Their rubric can be extended to describe the rationale for applying traditional psychiatric and positive interventions in clinical settings.

We expect that positive psychiatry will grow rapidly during the years and decades ahead. Under this umbrella, clinicians and educators would have somewhat different roles from those they currently have. Clinicians will evaluate not only psychopathology but also the levels of well-being and positive traits among their patients, and employ psychotherapeutic and behavioral (and possibly pharmacological and other biological) interventions to enhance those traits, focusing on improved well-being and recovery. When a greater emphasis is placed on positive outcomes, attributes, and strengths, the stigma against mental illness may be reduced, which may also help in recruiting trainees into psychiatry. Positive psychiatrists also will train their colleagues outside psychiatry in implementing similar interventions for people suffering from or at high risk for physical illnesses such as heart disease, metabolic disorders, and even some cancers.

If effective interventions to strengthen positive traits were provided to all psychiatric patients, considerably more people with serious mental illness might achieve recovery. Similarly, through well-designed and -implemented preventive strategies, positive psychiatry has the promise to improve health outcomes and reduce morbidity and mortality in the population. Instead of being narrowly defined as a medical subspecialty restricted to management of mental illnesses, psychiatry of the future will develop into a core component of the overall health care system. Psychiatrists will thus more explicitly reclaim their role as physicians in addition to their role as mental health professionals.

Combining Traditional Psychiatry With Positive Psychiatry

This book illustrates the various ways in which traditional and positive psychiatry approaches can be combined to help people with mental illnesses as well as other groups, such as people with physical illnesses and trainees in medicine or law. Later chapters in this book attempt to take the general framework we have articulated to the next level by providing specific and detailed case discussions that highlight the opportunities and dilemmas encountered in clinical work. Each case describes a patient or a setting and the context for seeking or providing help. Each individual's strengths and problems are discussed, and this is followed by a formulation of the situation, including these two elements. Next, the course of treatment and reflections on the care and interventions are provided.

Several questions arise in marrying traditional psychiatry with positive psychiatry:

1. Which patients benefit from traditional psychiatric approaches, which from positive interventions, and which from an appropriate combination of the two?

2. Which interventions work together synergistically and in what sequence?
3. How are traditional psychiatric and positive interventions best conceptualized when combined, and what is the best way to explain this to patients?
4. What are the best outcome measures to use to assess care that includes both symptom-reducing and positivity-enhancing interventions?

We hope you will read the cases, noticing the two main threads as they intertwine—traditional psychiatric treatments and positivity-enhancing interventions—and consider these important and clinically meaningful questions.

TAKE-HOME POINTS

- Positive psychiatry expands the perspective of traditional psychiatry beyond psychopathology to include the positive aspects of human life, including positive experiences, traits, and communities.

- Positive psychiatry is consistent with many traditions within the history of psychiatry. There is evidence of the positive being utilized within both psychotherapy and psychopharmacology.

- Positive psychiatry imagines a future in which positive interventions are used for improved outcomes in the field of mental health and also for enhancement in general medical care and beyond the clinic in education and organizational management.

REFERENCES

Adler MG, Fagley NS: Appreciation: individual differences in finding value and meaning as a unique predictor of subjective well-being. J Pers 73(1):79–114, 2005

Alarcon GM, Bowling NA, Khazon S: Great expectations: a meta-analytic examination of optimism and hope. Pers Individ Dif 54(7):821–827, 2013

Berry W: The pleasures of eating, in Cooking, Eating, Thinking: Transformative Philosophies of Food. Edited by Curtin D, Heldke L. Bloomington, Indiana University Press, 1992, pp 374–379

Bolier L, Haverman M, Westerhof GJ, et al: Positive psychology interventions: a meta-analysis of randomized controlled studies. BMC Public Health 13(1):119, 2013 23390882

Bretherton R, Ørner RJ: Positive psychology and psychotherapy: an existential approach, in Positive Psychology in Practice. Edited by Linley PA, Joseph S. New York, Wiley, 2004, pp 420–430

Brody S, Costa RM: Satisfaction (sexual, life, relationship, and mental health) is associated directly with penile-vaginal intercourse, but inversely with other sexual behavior frequencies. J Sex Med 6(7):1947–1954, 2009 19453891

Cappelletti S, Piacentino D, Sani G, et al: Caffeine: cognitive and physical performance enhancer or psychoactive drug? Curr Neuropharmacol 13(1):71–88, 2015 26074744

Carstensen LL, Fung HH, Charles ST: Socioemotional selectivity theory and the regulation of emotion in the second half of life. Motiv Emot 27(2):103–123, 2003

Cheavens JS, Feldman DB, Gum A, et al: Hope therapy in a community sample: a pilot investigation. Social Indicators Research 77(1):61–78, 2006

Chodorow NJ: The psychoanalytic vision of Hans Loewald. Int J Psychoanal 84 (Pt 4):897–913, 2003 13678496

Cooney G, Dwan K, Mead G: Exercise for depression. JAMA 311(23):2432–2433, 2014 24938566

Crews DJ, Lochbaum MR, Landers DM: Aerobic physical activity effects on psychological well-being in low-income Hispanic children. Percept Mot Skills 98(1):319–324, 2004 15058892

Davison SL, Bell RJ, LaChina M, et al: The relationship between self-reported sexual satisfaction and general well-being in women. J Sex Med 6(10):2690–2697, 2009 19817981

Dyrbye LN, Thomas MR, Massie FS, et al: Burnout and suicidal ideation among US medical students: medical student burnout and suicidal ideation. Ann Intern Med 149(5):334-341, 2008

Eckleberry-Hunt J, Lick D, Boura J, et al: An exploratory study of resident burnout and wellness. Acad Med 84(2):269–277, 2009 19174684

Emmons RA, McCullough ME: Counting blessings versus burdens: an experimental investigation of gratitude and subjective well-being in daily life. J Pers Soc Psychol 84(2):377–389, 2003 12585811

Erikson EH: Identity and the life cycle: selected papers. Psychol Issues 1:1–171, 1959

Fowler RD, Seligman ME, Koocher GP: The APA 1998 Annual Report. Am Psychol 54(8):537–568, 1999

Freud S: The Joke and Its Relation to the Unconscious (1905). Translated by Crick J. New York, Penguin, 2003

Freud S: The relation of the poet to day-dreaming (1908), in Character and Culture. Edited by Rieff P. New York, Collier Books, 1972, pp 34–43

Freud S: The theme of the three caskets (1913), in The Standard Edition of the Complete Psychological Works of Sigmund Freud, Vol 12. Translated and edited by Strachey J. London, Hogarth Press, 1958, pp 291–301

Freud S: The Moses of Michelangelo (1914), in The Standard Edition of the Complete Psychological Works of Sigmund Freud, Vol 8. Translated and edited by Strachey J. London, Hogarth Press, 1955, pp 291–301

Gabbard GO: Textbook of Psychotherapeutic Treatments. Washington, DC, American Psychiatric Publishing, 2009

Gallagher MW, Lopez SJ: Positive expectancies and mental health: identifying the unique contributions of hope and optimism. J Posit Psychol 4(6):548–556, 2009

Gander F, Proyer RT, Ruch W, et al: Strength-based positive interventions: further evidence for their potential in enhancing well-being and alleviating depression. J Happiness Stud 14(4):1241–1259, 2013

Gill MM: Ego psychology and psychotherapy. Psychoanal Q 20(1):62–71, 1951 14834272

Gillham JE, Reivich KJ, Jaycox LH, et al: Prevention of depressive symptoms in school children: two-year follow-up. Psychol Sci 6(6):343–351, 1995

Gillham JE, Shatte AJ, Reivich KJ, Seligman ME: Optimism, pessimism, and explanatory style, in Optimism and Pessimism: Implications for Theory, Research, and Practice. Edited by Chang EC. Washington, DC, American Psychological Association, 2001, pp 53–75

Gillham JE, Reivich KJ, Freres DR, et al: School-based prevention of depressive symptoms: a randomized controlled study of the effectiveness and specificity of the Penn Resiliency Program. J Consult Clin Psychol 75(1):9–19, 2007 17295559

Griffiths RR, Richards WA, McCann U, et al: Psilocybin can occasion mystical-type experiences having substantial and sustained personal meaning and spiritual significance. Psychopharmacology (Berl) 187(3):268–283, discussion 284–292, 2006 16826400

Griffiths RR, Richards W, Johnson M, et al: Mystical-type experiences occasioned by psilocybin mediate the attribution of personal meaning and spiritual significance 14 months later. J Psychopharmacol 22(6):621–632, 2008 18593735

Griffiths RR, Johnson MW, Carducci MA, et al: Psilocybin produces substantial and sustained decreases in depression and anxiety in patients with life-threatening cancer: a randomized double-blind trial. J Psychopharmacol 30(12):1181–1197, 2016 27909165

Heller T, Hsieh K, Rimmer JH: Attitudinal and psychosocial outcomes of a fitness and health education program on adults with Down syndrome. American Journal on Mental Retardation 109(2):175–185, 2004

Herzberg PY, Glaesmer H, Hoyer J: Separating optimism and pessimism: a robust psychometric analysis of the revised Life Orientation Test (LOT-R). Psychol Assess 18(4):433–438, 2006 17154764

Holmberg D, Blair KL, Phillips M: Women's sexual satisfaction as a predictor of well-being in same-sex versus mixed-sex relationships. J Sex Res 47(1):1–11, 2010 19381998

Hooghe M: Is sexual well-being part of subjective well-being? An empirical analysis of Belgian (Flemish) survey data using an extended well-being scale. J Sex Res 49(2–3):264–273, 2012 21298588

James W: The Varieties of Religious Experience. New York, New American Library, 2017

Jeste DV, Palmer BW (eds): Positive Psychiatry: A Clinical Handbook. Washington, DC, American Psychiatric Association, 2015

Jeste DV, Depp CA, Vahia IV: Successful cognitive and emotional aging. World Psychiatry 9(2):78–84, 2010 20671889

Jeste DV, Savla GN, Thompson WK, et al: Association between older age and more successful aging: critical role of resilience and depression. Am J Psychiatry 170(2):188–196, 2013 23223917

Jeste DV, Palmer BW, Rettew DC, et al: Positive psychiatry: its time has come. J Clin Psychiatry 76(6):675–683, 2015 26132670

Jeste DV, Palmer BW, Saks ER: Why we need positive psychiatry for schizophrenia and other psychotic disorders. Schizophr Bull 43(2):227–229, 2017 28399307

Kashdan TB, Uswatte G, Julian T: Gratitude and hedonic and eudaimonic well-being in Vietnam War veterans. Behav Res Ther 44(2):177–199, 2006 16389060

Kendler KS, Liu XQ, Gardner CO, et al: Dimensions of religiosity and their relationship to lifetime psychiatric and substance use disorders. Am J Psychiatry 160(3):496–503, 2003 12611831

Laumann EO, Paik A, Glasser DB, et al: A cross-national study of subjective sexual well-being among older women and men: findings from the Global Study of Sexual Attitudes and Behaviors. Arch Sex Behav 35(2):145–161, 2006 16752118

Layous K, Nelson SK, Lyubomirsky S: What is the optimal way to deliver a positive activity intervention? The case of writing about one's best possible selves. Journal of Happiness Studies 14(2):635–654, 2013

Linley A, Joseph S, Harrington S, Wood AM: Positive psychology: past, present, and (possible) future. Journal of Positive Psychology 1(1);3-16, 2006

Loewald HW: On the therapeutic action of psycho-analysis. Int J Psychoanal 41:16–33, 1960 14417912

Macht M, Dettmer D: Everyday mood and emotions after eating a chocolate bar or an apple. Appetite 46(3):332–336, 2006 16546294

Maslow AH: Toward a Psychology of Being (1962). New York, Simon & Schuster, 2013

McCabe SE, West BT, Morales M, et al: Does early onset of non-medical use of prescription drugs predict subsequent prescription drug abuse and dependence? Results from a national study. Addiction 102(12):1920–1930, 2007 17916222

McCray LW, Cronholm PF, Bogner HR, et al: Resident physician burnout: is there hope? Fam Med 40(9):626, 2008

McCullough ME: Savoring life, past and present: explaining what hope and gratitude share in common. Psychological Inquiry 13(4):302–304, 2002

McLafferty CL Jr, Wetzstein CJ, Hunter GR: Resistance training is associated with improved mood in healthy older adults. Percept Mot Skills 98 (3 Pt 1):947–957, 2004 15209311

Meyer PS, Johnson DP, Parks A, et al: Positive living: a pilot study of group positive psychotherapy for people with schizophrenia. J Posit Psychol 7(3):239–248, 2012

Michener W, Rozin P: Pharmacological versus sensory factors in the satiation of chocolate craving. Physiol Behav 56(3):419–422, 1994

Mitchell J, Stanimirovic R, Klein B, Vella-Brodrick D: A randomised controlled trial of a self-guided internet intervention promoting well-being. Computers in Human Behavior 25(3):749–760, 2009

Mongrain M, Anselmo-Matthews T: Do positive psychology exercises work? A replication of Seligman et al (2005): J Clin Psychol 68(4):382–389, 2012 24469930

Olfson M, Blanco C, Liu SM, et al: National trends in the office-based treatment of children, adolescents, and adults with antipsychotics. Arch Gen Psychiatry 69(12):1247–1256, 2012 22868273

Park N, Peterson C: Moral competence and character strengths among adolescents: the development and validation of the Values in Action Inventory of Strengths for Youth. J Adolesc 29(6):891–909, 2006 16766025

Park N, Peterson C, Seligman ME: Strengths of character and well-being. J Soc Clin Psychol 23(5):603–619, 2004

Park N, Peterson C, Seligman MEP: Character strengths in fifty-four nations and the fifty US states. J Posit Psychol 1(3):118–129, 2006

Peters ML, Flink IK, Boersma K, Linton SJ: Manipulating optimism: can imagining a best possible self be used to increase positive future expectancies? Journal of Positive Psychology 5(3):204–211, 2010

Peterson C, Seligman ME: Character Strengths and Virtues: A Handbook and Classification, Vol 1. New York, Oxford University Press, 2004

Peterson C, Semmel A, Von Baeyer C, et al: The Attributional Style Questionnaire. Cognit Ther Res 6(3):287–299, 1982

Proyer RT, Ruch W, Buschor C: Testing strengths-based interventions: a preliminary study on the effectiveness of a program targeting curiosity, gratitude, hope, humor, and zest for enhancing life satisfaction. J Happiness Stud 14(1):275–292, 2013

Quinlan D, Swain N, Vella-Brodrick DA: Character strengths interventions: building on what we know for improved outcomes. J Happiness Stud 13(6):1145–1163, 2012

Reed J, Ones DS: The effect of acute aerobic exercise on positive activated affect: a meta-analysis. Psychol Sport Exerc 7(5):477–514, 2006

Resnick SG, Rosenheck RA: Recovery and positive psychology: parallel themes and potential synergies. Psychiatr Serv 57(1):120–122, 2006 16399972

Rettew D: Child Temperament: New Thinking About the Boundary Between Traits and Illness. New York, WW Norton, 2013

Rockland LH: Supportive Therapy. New York, Basic Books, 2003

Rosenthal RN, Westreich LM: Cosmetic psychopharmacology: drugs that enhance well-being, performance, and creativity, in Clinical Addiction Psychiatry. Edited by Brizer D, Castaneda R. New York, Cambridge University Press, 2010, pp 72–87

Rust T, Diessner R, Reade L: Strengths only or strengths and relative weaknesses? A preliminary study. J Psychol 143(5):465–476, 2009 19943398

Seligman ME: The president's address. Am Psychol 54:559–562, 1999

Seligman ME: Authentic Happiness: Using the New Positive Psychology to Realize Your Potential for Lasting Fulfillment. New York, Simon & Schuster, 2004

Seligman ME: The Optimistic Child: A Proven Program to Safeguard Children Against Depression and Build Lifelong Resilience. Boston, MA, Houghton Mifflin Harcourt, 2007

Seligman ME, Csikszentmihalyi M: Positive psychology: an introduction, in Flow and the Foundations of Positive Psychology: The Collected Works of Mihaly Csikszentmihalyi. Dordrecht, Springer Netherlands, 2014, pp 279–298

Seligman M, Steen T, Park N, Peterson C: Positive psychology progress. Am Psychol 60(5):410–421, 2005

Sheldon KM, King L: Why positive psychology is necessary. Am Psychol 56(3):216–217, 2001 11315247

Sheldon KM, Lyubomirsky S: How to increase and sustain positive emotion: the effects of expressing gratitude and visualizing best possible selves. J Posit Psychol 1(2):73–82, 2006

Siqueland LR, Barber JP: Supportive-expressive psychotherapy, in Comprehensive Handbook of Psychotherapy, Vol 1: Psychodynamic/Object Relations. Edited by Kaslow FW, Magnavita JJ. New York, Wiley, 2002, pp 183–206

Slade M: Mental illness and well-being: the central importance of positive psychology and recovery approaches. BMC Health Serv Res 10:26, 2010 20102609

Smith ME, Farah MJ: Are prescription stimulants "smart pills"? The epidemiology and cognitive neuroscience of prescription stimulant use by normal healthy individuals. Psychol Bull 137(5):717–741, 2011 21859174

Snodgrass J, LeBaron P: National Survey on Drug Use and Health: CAI Specifications for Programming, English Version. Rockville, MD, Substance Abuse and Mental Health Services Administration, 2008

Snyder CR: Hope theory: rainbows in the mind. Psychol Inq 13(4):249–275, 2002

Snyder CR, Lopez SJ, Pedrotti JT: Positive Psychology: The Scientific and Practical Explorations of Human Strengths, 2nd Edition. Thousand Oaks, CA, Sage, 2011

Stein DJ: Positive mental health: a note of caution. World Psychiatry 11(2):107–109, 2012a 22654942

Stein DJ: Psychopharmacological enhancement: a conceptual framework. Philos Ethics Humanit Med 7:5, 2012b 22244084

Stubbs B, Vancampfort D, Rosenbaum S, et al: An examination of the anxiolytic effects of exercise for people with anxiety and stress-related disorders: a meta-analysis. Psychiatry Res 249:102–108, 2017 28088704

Studerus E, Kometer M, Hasler F, et al: Acute, subacute and long-term subjective effects of psilocybin in healthy humans: a pooled analysis of experimental studies. J Psychopharmacol 25(11):1434–1452, 2011 20855349

Summers RF, Lord JA: Positivity in supportive and psychodynamic therapy, in Positive Psychiatry: A Clinical Handbook. Edited by Jeste DV, Palmer BW. Washington, DC, American Psychiatric Association, 2015, pp 167–192

Vaillant GE: The Wisdom of the Ego. Cambridge, MA, Harvard University Press, 1993

Vaillant GE: Aging Well: Surprising Guideposts to a Happier Life From the Landmark Study of Adult Development. New York, Little, Brown, 2008

Watkins PC, Woodward K, Stone T, Kolts RL: Gratitude and happiness: development of a measure of gratitude, and relationships with subjective well-being. Social Behavior and Personality 31(5):431–451, 2003

West CP, Dyrbye LN, Erwin PJ, et al: Interventions to prevent and reduce physician burnout: a systematic review and meta-analysis. Lancet 388(10057):2272–2281, 2016

Wood AM, Joseph S, Lloyd J, et al: Gratitude influences sleep through the mechanism of pre-sleep cognitions. J Psychosom Res 66(1):43–48, 2009 19073292

Wood AM, Froh JJ, Geraghty AW: Gratitude and well-being: a review and theoretical integration. Clin Psychol Rev 30(7):890–905, 2010 20451313

Yalom ID: Existential Psychotherapy. New York, Basic Books, 1980

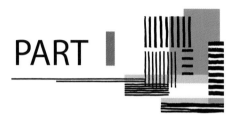

PART I

Mental Health Care

Section Editors:
Richard F. Summers, M.D.
Dilip V. Jeste, M.D.

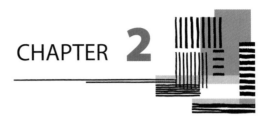

CHAPTER 2

A Family- and Wellness-Based Approach to Child Emotional-Behavioral Problems

David C. Rettew, M.D.

Editors' Introduction

This chapter describes a young girl with social anxiety whose treatment focuses on health, wellness, and positivity. The interventions are very accessible for the girl and her parents and represent a broad focus of assessment and intervention. The treatment approach is remarkably nonstigmatizing for this family. The focus is rather pragmatic in that a number of interventions are discussed and the family is able to move forward with some more than others; this is accepted and indeed expected by the psychiatrist. The approach has a light touch that makes it accessible to the family and contrasts with what the experience of psychopharmacology or more intensive behavioral approaches might be like for them.

SUMMARY

This case example describes a 7-year-old girl who presents with increasing anxiety and reluctance to go to school in the context of a number of family and social challenges. From a conventional psychiatric perspective, the case looks like a typical one in which cognitive-behavioral therapy and/or medication would be considered. However, an enhanced assessment from a positive psychiatry perspective reveals a number of additional avenues for intervention, such as encouraging musical training and mindfulness in addition to directly addressing parental psychopathology and parenting practices. The chapter provides a practical example for how a wellness plan can be designed and implemented as part of routine practice for all patients. This patient responds very well to a number of wellness and health promotion activities and begins to have a much more positive developmental trajectory with these efforts.

Positive psychiatry principles can be readily applied to children and adolescents (Rettew 2015). The case in this chapter—a composite of a 7-year-old girl who suffers from anxiety—showcases a number of ways in which the clinician can use positive psychiatry to add important elements to both the assessment and the treatment plan while still working within the general framework of standard outpatient treatment. Some of the case information will be presented sequentially to demonstrate how an assessment procedure that is family and wellness based leads to treatment avenues that might otherwise be overlooked. Many of the core principles and procedures described here can be thought of not only as positive psychiatry per se but also as belonging to other models of care such as the Vermont Family Based Approach as developed and described by Hudziak and Ivanova (2016).

Person

Haley is a 7-year-old girl who lives with her biological parents and younger brother. She presents with a long history of anxiety that is increasingly causing problems at home, at school, and in her peer relationships. Haley is in second grade at her local public elementary school. Her mother previously worked in the medical records division of a local hospital but now stays at home with the children. The father is currently working in the information technology department of a large company. Haley arrives with her mother to the initial appointment with a child psychiatrist. Haley initially sits quietly and very close to her mother on the couch, but with some prompting she walks over to the dollhouse in the office and begins playing. When asked, Haley admits to feeling nervous or anxious quite a bit but has a difficult time identifying exactly what she is afraid of, other than not liking to be alone. When the psychiatrist asks about spending some time with just Haley, the mother replies, "I don't think she'll go for it, but you're welcome to try." Indeed, Haley shakes her head at the idea and insists that the interview take place with everyone present in the room.

Haley was the product of an uncomplicated pregnancy and delivery. She was born full-term and met her developmental milestones on time. Her mother reports that, temperamentally, Haley was somewhat shy and reserved as a toddler. When Haley was 2 years old, her mother attempted to return to employment. Haley became so distraught at being dropped off at a day care center, however, after two tries they gave up and decided to keep Haley at home. The transition to kindergarten was also a struggle, and Haley often misses several school days per month because of vague aches and pains that do not have a clear cause.

The mother adamantly denies any history of trauma or abuse for Haley, although she does wonder, given her daughter's extreme distress when they have tried to "push her too far to do things," whether such demands could be considered traumatic for her. Haley does have two close friends whom she sees outside of school but prefers that they come to her house rather than the other way around. Haley enjoys drawing, and the parents have provided her with a lot of art supplies to encourage this. She does not participate in organized sports or clubs, and a couple of previous attempts to try things like group swim lessons or team soccer have not gone well. The mother also denies any history of diagnosed mental illness in the family but states that she "was kind of the same way" when she was a child.

One source of conflict at home is around sleeping. Haley continues to need her mother to be present in her room for her to fall asleep. Later in the night, Haley often awakens and gets into her parents' bed. Haley's mother does not mind this, but her father has become increasingly irritated with this behavior and now sometimes moves into Haley's room to sleep when this happens. This struggle reflects a larger divide in parental approach in which the father has become more detached in his interactions with Haley as he finds himself increasingly frustrated with her level of dependence. The mother states that because of Haley's needs at night, she and her husband have not left the children with a babysitter in several years.

Haley also can be a picky eater and does not like to try new foods. The parents initially tried to "force" her to eat the same meals that they were having, but have since moved to giving her a rotation of about four different combinations that she is willing to eat.

After Haley's difficulty coping with the transition to kindergarten, her mother found a private therapist in town, who saw Haley approximately every other week for nearly a year. The mother isn't quite sure what happened in the therapy, but much of the therapy was play based. No official diagnosis was given, but the mother remembers being told that themes of anxiety did emerge in her play and that the therapist attempted to work with those feelings. Although Haley enjoyed these sessions, the family eventually discontinued them because of the cost and lack of substantive improvement. After a number of school absences in the first grade, Haley's teacher brought up the question of an anxiety disorder and suggested a formal evaluation. Haley's father initially resisted this recommendation because of his concern that a doctor would just want to "drug" his daughter. However, with the continued school absences and Haley's difficulty coping both academically and socially, the parents finally agreed to this evaluation.

During the interview, Haley reports some worrying that "something bad" will happen to her mother, but she is vague about how often and intense these feelings are. Her mother notes that this concern comes up occasionally and that Haley sometimes describes nightmares of being left alone. More often, however, Haley seems "just nervous and timid" at baseline without articulating a lot of specific fears to the parents. When Haley is not being challenged, Haley's mood is generally good, and, indeed, she can be quite lively when interacting with her parents and close friends. Recently, however, Haley has begun to make some negative comments about herself. For example, when a friend of hers came to the house recently to play, Haley noticed that her friend was wearing her soccer uniform and then told her friend, "I'm not very good at sports."

From the existing information, there is much to suggest that Haley suffers from separation anxiety disorder. The presence of these difficulties at a very early age in the absence of specific stressors or trauma also suggests the possibility that there is a strong temperamental component to her behavior. Her history is quite consistent with Kagan's (1994) definition of *behavioral inhibition*, which he describes as a temperamental disposition to being reserved and withdrawn when confronted with new people and situations.

The history also suggests that her struggles are beginning to snowball toward greater and greater impairment that, if unchecked, could lead to possible mood disorders and further isolation. As Haley's peers develop new interests and expand their social skills, Haley's anxiety is impeding her ability to undertake many of the expected developmental tasks for her age group. This gap between her and her peers is starting to be noticed by Haley and is likely to negatively impact her self-esteem, which, in turn, can perpetuate this vicious cycle even further.

Many clinicians at this point would conclude that Haley's emotional-behavioral problems are significant enough to require formal treatment and would be considering one or both of the two main forms of psychiatric interventions, namely psychotherapy and pharmacotherapy. The fact that she has already had a course of individual psychotherapy without major benefit might prompt many psychiatrists to consider a trial of a selective serotonin reuptake inhibitor such as fluoxetine or sertraline. Alternatively, or in conjunction with pharmacotherapy, a course of cognitive-behavioral therapy might also be recommended to help Haley identify maladaptive thoughts that might be contributing to her anxiety and to help her learn specific coping skills.

ADDITIONAL ASSESSMENT FROM A POSITIVE PSYCHIATRY APPROACH

Based on the adage that "when you're a hammer, everything looks like a nail," it is critical to point out that the success of using positive psychiatry principles in treatment depends on the ability to collect good information about wellness and health promotion during the assessment. An evaluation that focuses exclusively on a patient's symptoms and skills deficits will very likely rely on medications and individual therapy alone as interventions. In contrast, an evaluation that investigates the patient's and the family's strengths and engagement across multiple domains of positive psychiatry and wellness allows for a number of additional avenues for intervention that can improve the odds not only for symptom improvement but also for an overall better quality of life. The following subsections present some other information that might be collected according to a positive psychiatry model that could be used toward an expanded formulation.

Parental Psychopathology

Preliminary data suggest that the standard family history questions miss approximately *half* of existing parental psychopathology (Basoglu et al. 2014). Given the known benefit to children of assessing and treating parental psychopathology (Siegenthaler et al. 2012), clinicians should consider a more rigorous screening of parents—not so much in the service of arriving at a more accurate diagnosis for the child but primarily to identify additional treatments and supports for the parents themselves that might in turn benefit the patient and the entire family.

Prior to the appointment, the psychiatrist in this case asks the parents to fill out not only the broad-based Child Behavior Checklist about Haley but also rating scales for themselves and each other, using the Adult Behavior Checklist and the Adult Self-Report (Achenbach and Rescorla 2001, 2003). The results of these assessments reveal that Haley's mother scores in the clinical range for anxious/depressed problems herself and the father has been drinking alcohol excessively. Neither parent is receiving any treatment at this time.

In light of this new information, it seems quite likely that the mother's own level of anxiety may be contributing to a cycle of overprotectiveness that, while well meaning, is further limiting Haley's opportunities to address and overcome her anxiety and causing Haley to feel more isolated and more deviant from her peers (Lieb et al. 2000). Both the mother's anxiety and the father's drinking are also impacting their ability to provide the level of positive energy and warmth that has been shown to be a critical factor for positive child development (Patterson 1982).

The clinician realizes that a large part of the success of any kind of cognitive-behavioral program for Haley will depend on the parents' abilities to carry out treatment recommendations outside of the sessions. Decreased anxiety in the mother can be expected to result in decreased anxiety in her daughter. Also, by controlling his alcohol use, the father may be able to become more involved in family interactions and to be a fully present and effective parent.

Including the Whole Family

Recognizing the need to have a positive relationship with all family members before behavior change is likely to occur, the psychiatrist strongly encourages the father to come in and give his perspective. When he does, he corroborates much of what his wife has reported but does add some additional elements. He admits that he has been getting increasingly frustrated with his daughter's anxiety, although he knows he should not become angry. He also states that he feels that Haley needs to be "pushed" a little more but that his wife does not agree. Seeing Haley struggle has been difficult for him and has made him feel "incompetent" as a father. In trying to cope with this shame and disappointment, he reports that he has been drinking more and engaging less with his wife and daughter. The psychiatrist validates these feelings and behaviors but points out how they may run counter to Haley's positive development. He then invites and strongly urges the father to attend as many future appointments as possible.

Positive Traits

In addition to asking the parents about Haley's challenges, the psychiatrist encourages the parents to talk about Haley's strengths and helps them by showing them a list from the VIA Survey of Character Strengths (http://www.viacharacter.org). They identify a number of strengths in many of the five core domains of wisdom and knowledge, courage, humanity, justice, and temperance. The specific traits that are particularly prominent in Haley include creativity, honesty, kindness, and fairness. The parents visibly brighten when discussing these positive aspects of Haley's personality (as most parents do when given the opportunity to say nice things about their child), and the psychiatrist challenges them to think of ways that these traits can be utilized in the treatment plan.

Domains of Wellness

As shown in Table 2–1, a number of aspects of wellness should be assessed at the family level and incorporated into an intervention plan. All of these domains have been supported from research (Hudziak 2008; Jeste et al. 2015).

TABLE 2–1. Wellness plan example for Haley

Domain	Current status	Current status rating (deficient, adequate, exemplary)	Priority for change (low, medium, high)	Specific initial goals
Physical activity and exercise	Little structured or unstructured activity family-wide	Deficient	High	Daily physical activity; family to learn/do one specific activity together
Music and arts	Draws and paints but no musical training	Deficient	Medium	Parents to research violin lessons
Mindfulness	No formal instruction	Deficient	Medium	Parent and child to begin twice-daily mindfulness with smartphone app
Screen time	1–2 hours per day with occasional inappropriate content	Adequate	Low	Father to limit access to inappropriate content; screen time linked to other wellness activities
Sleep	Duration adequate but sleeping in parents' bed	Deficient	Medium	Design behavioral plan to encourage increased time in own bed
Nutrition	Adequate nutrition but limited food choices	Adequate	Low	Introduce one new nutritious food per week

TABLE 2–1. Wellness plan example for Haley (*continued*)

Domain	Current status	Current status rating (deficient, adequate, exemplary)	Priority for change (low, medium, high)	Specific initial goals
Charity	No current activities	Deficient	Low	After other new things introduced, family to consider return to church community
Hydration	Drinks at meals but not otherwise	Deficient	Low	Drink an additional 3 cups of water per day
Positive parenting	Some limit setting but warmth and positive experiences compromised	Deficient	High	Encourage parental self-care; include parental guidance recommendations in counseling sessions
Parental psychopathology	Both parents screen positive for possible psychopathology, and neither treated	Deficient	High	Referral for parents' own full evaluation and treatment

Haley's psychiatrist discovers that the girl's family, like most families, is doing pretty well in some areas while struggling in others. With regard to *nutrition*, the family tends to serve healthy choices for meals and limits their consumption of less healthy snacks and desserts. As mentioned, Haley's food repertoire is limited, but what she does eat is nutritionally sound. In the area of *physical activity and exercise*, Haley has become significantly less active as she has withdrawn from sports teams. Neither of her parents currently engages in regular exercise either. *Sleep* is also a challenge for Haley, as she cannot fall asleep on her own and wakes up during the night to go into her parents' room. The mother's willingness to accept these behaviors has resulted in less conflict at night and longer sleep durations for Haley, but the father does not see this as a long-term solution. In the area of *music and arts*, Haley does indeed like to spend time drawing and expressed interest in learning how to play a violin once after her mother talked about playing one as a child.

When asked about *screen time*, the parents state that Haley enjoys seeing some shows and movies for about 1–2 hours per day. They do not permit her to look at screens for long periods of time and acknowledge that Haley rarely fights these limits. On a few occasions, Haley has joined her father while he watched television and has seen some violent content that has frightened her and "given her nightmares."

The family used to attend a Christian church but stopped going when it became difficult to drop off Haley for Sunday school prior to services. Since then, their *participation in charitable activities and giving back to others* has diminished, although the parents strongly believe in this principle. Regarding *mindfulness*, Haley's mother states that she sometimes tries to help Haley take deep breaths when she is upset but reports that they have never attempted a more systematic approach. Finally, in the area of *hydration*, Haley readily drinks juice or milk at mealtimes but does not drink much water between these times.

Overall, the findings from the assessment of these domains of positive psychiatry do not necessarily refute the original formulation but substantially enrich it. The untreated parental psychopathology and low levels of engagement in several areas of wellness represent important untapped sources of potential improvement. Furthermore, a review of Haley's strengths leads the clinician to consider some areas that can be targeted for promoting her personal growth. For example, Haley's kindness could help in motivating her to become involved in projects or activities that give back to others, whereas her creativity and interest in music could help in encouraging her to engage in music lessons and perhaps eventually a youth orchestra.

In trying to summarize the information to the parents, the psychiatrist begins by stating that Haley seems like a wonderful little girl who is lucky to have two loving and supportive parents but who is also struggling with significant anxiety that is increasingly holding her back. The clinician explains that the child's struggles meet criteria for separation anxiety disorder and that she is beginning to show some signs of depression. Haley's difficulties have arisen out of a combination of genetic and environmental factors that often conspire together to create cycles that can reinforce initial predispositions. The good news, however, is that there exist multiple entry points to help break and even reverse this cycle through a multimodal family-based approach that incorporates not only more traditional psychiatric interventions but also evidence-based treatment based on principles of positive psychiatry and wellness.

INTERVENTIONS

The incorporation of positive psychiatry domains in the assessment allows for an augmented treatment plan that directly targets these domains. Whether these areas *replace* (at least at first) the more traditional interventions of individual psychotherapy and psychopharmacology or are used *adjunctively* depends on a number of factors, including the severity of the problems, the wishes of the patient and parents, and the judgment of the clinician.

These decisions are optimally discussed in a full-length feedback session in which the clinician shares with the parents the results of the evaluation and scores on the various rating scales, and assesses the parents' overall emotional strengths and weaknesses, degree of involvement in wellness activities, and strength of routines and wellness activities. At the same time, the clinician is trying to determine the family's readiness level to engage in behavior change and, if need be, attempting to motivate the family further along the stages of change. A more formal protocol for this session is the Family Assessment and Feedback Intervention (Ivanova 2013).

When the clinician is presenting assessment results, it is important not to blame parents for the child's behavioral problems. Some parents arrive at a child psychiatry session already burdened with a great deal of self-blame, and others can be quick to become defensive, resulting in disengagement from the treatment process. Thus, it is often critical for the clinician to convey his or her appreciation for how difficult raising children can be, especially when both the child and the parents are struggling with psychopathology.

Organizing and prioritizing the many aspects of positive psychiatry can often be augmented through the use of a written wellness plan that becomes a working document for the whole family. Table 2–1 is an example of one as it relates to Haley's case, but clinicians can devise their own based on what works best for their particular clinic and patients. Journals or even smartphone apps can also be used to help families remember and track progress.

The precise structure of positive psychiatry–oriented treatment can vary. In one format, the psychiatrist himself or herself meets with the family at regular intervals (every week or every other week) to review the wellness plan, offer parental guidance, provide evidence-based psychotherapy, and monitor progress. These elements can occur in the same session in which pharmacological treatment takes place. From a Vermont Family Based Approach perspective (Hudziak and Ivanova 2016), the psychiatrist would then be considered to be performing all three roles of family-based treatment: the family coach (who works on the wellness plan), the focused family coach (who provides evidence-based psychotherapy), and the family-based psychiatrist (who coordinates the team, provides medical oversight, and does the psychopharmacological treatment if indicated). Generally, appointments that encompass all of these elements would need to take 45–50 minutes each. Although there are many advantages of consolidating these roles within one person, it is also important to consider the practical limitations of such a physician-intensive treatment. An alternative might be for a nonphysician therapist and counselor to serve as the family coach and/or focused family coach after receiving some additional training in a wellness- and family-based model. Under these circumstances, the psychiatrist collaborates with the other team members and is then able to see the patient and family less frequently and for a shorter duration. Notably, the now-ubiquitous 15-minute "med checks" are not generally conducive to the treatment model described here.

In Hayley's case, the psychiatrist chooses to do the family coaching and positive psychiatry interventions himself. In the feedback session, he reviews the collected data, including the parents' mental health rating scales. The psychiatrist empathizes with the natural reaction to want to protect a more anxious child but proposes that the mother's level of anxiety is leading to some overprotection that is well meaning but possibly exacerbating Haley's anxiety and isolation. Meanwhile, the father's drinking and his increased irritability with the family situation are preventing him from being a more positive force in his daughter's treatment. After some discussion, the child psychiatrist and family decide to hold off on starting a medication and begin with family-oriented treatment that maximizes the use of positive psychiatry principles. The specifics of this plan are laid out in the following subsections.

Positive Parenting

The psychiatrist and family together identify a cycle in which Haley's behavior difficulties are increasing the stress load on both parents, which in turn is making both of them feel like they have "run out of gas," thus further reducing their frequency of positive interactions with Haley. Although the parents recognize that Haley often responds best to warm, supportive encouragement, their own negative emotional states quickly propel them to "go to the dark side" and become irritable and impatient. The psychiatrist provides some education to illustrate just how important parental warmth is for children and begins to strategize with the parents about ways they can enhance this. By encouraging the parents to remember Haley's many positive traits that they have helped nurture, the psychiatrist reminds them of some of their successes. The psychiatrist also encourages Haley's mother to do some things away from the family to help replenish her own parental reserve.

Education is also given about the difficult balance that parents try to achieve between protecting and overprotecting their children (Rettew 2013). The psychiatrist discusses how overprotectiveness with a more anxious child like Haley can lead to fewer opportunities for her to confront and eventually overcome her fears. Haley's parents are asked to begin monitoring these parental behaviors more closely by writing in a journal. With the psychiatrist's help, they begin to prepare for the resistance that might come from Haley when they encourage her to attempt some of the new activities proposed in the wellness plan.

Parental Psychopathology

Haley's parents are shown their results on the Adult Self-Report and Adult Behavior Checklist that indicate the possibility that each of them struggles with his or her own psychopathology. The psychiatrist praises their honesty in filling out the rating scales and their courage to acknowledge these challenges. He tries to normalize their difficulties by discussing the dimensional nature of psychopathology and commenting that the vast majority of people struggle, at least from time to time, with significant levels of psychiatric symptoms (Schaefer et al. 2017). He also provides education about the genetic influence on anxiety and alcohol problems, which, perhaps ironically, helps them both feel less to blame personally about their own and their daughter's symptoms. After this discussion, the psychiatrist refers both parents to an adult psychiatrist for further evaluation and possible treatment.

Physical Activity and Exercise

In discussions with the psychiatrist, the parents express a lot of pessimism about Haley's ability to restart a team sport without this becoming a major battleground. They agree it is an important long-term goal but decide to begin with a physical activity that Haley might be able to do with her parents and without a lot of crowds and people. With Haley's input, they decide on cross-country skiing at a nearby park for the winter and jogging in the warmer months. Haley is also given a device to wear that keeps track of her daily steps.

Music and Arts

Haley previously expressed interest in learning the violin, and her mother used to play violin as a child. The psychiatrist urges the mother to take out the instrument and let Haley explore it. They also set a goal for the mother to find places where Haley might begin to take lessons.

Mindfulness

In one of the follow-up sessions with Haley and her parents, the psychiatrist shows them several smartphone apps and Web sites where free guided mindfulness sessions can be found. They find one Haley likes and do a short session together in the appointment. They agree to begin each appointment with a session like this and set a goal for Haley and a parent to practice mindfulness at least twice a day.

Screen Time

The psychiatrist provides some education about what is known about the effects of excessive screen time and exposure to content that is not at Haley's developmental level. He reviews the current guidelines from the American Academy of Pediatrics (Council on Communications and Media 2016). The father agrees to prohibit Haley from watching inappropriate content, particularly things that might scare her. The parents also agree that Haley will begin to *earn* her screen time by doing other activities such as exercise and reading.

Sleep

In a subsequent appointment, the mother expresses some concern that some of the new activities being encouraged for Haley are going to be met with increased anxiety. The mother wonders whether trying additionally to get Haley to sleep in her own bed at the same time is asking too much. The father takes part in these discussions and would like to see Haley's nightly migration to the parents' bed stop, but he agrees that this could be difficult as other aspects of the wellness plan are implemented. They agree to monitor this behavior for now, with a goal to begin instituting the "camping out" sleep training program, in which a parent gradually moves farther and farther away from the child as she falls asleep (Price et al. 2012), at some point soon. The psychiatrist also suggests that it might help for the father to begin taking a more active role in Haley's bedtime routine and that this could actually facilitate the transition to Haley being able to get to sleep in her own room.

Nutrition

Although the parents would like to see Haley accept a wider number of foods, they find this area to be of lower priority given the fact that she does enjoy foods from all major food groups and is growing normally. They decide as an initial plan that they will continue to introduce and encourage new foods regularly but will not push the issue at this point.

Charity

The family used to participate in a local church and stopped going because of difficulties related to dropping off Haley for child care and Sunday school. Both parents miss this community, which often was engaged in efforts to help those who are less fortunate. The psychiatrist notes that Haley's character strengths include kindness and fairness, which would well be harnessed in efforts to help other people. However, the parents also acknowledge that any reintroduction to the church would need to proceed gradually.

Hydration

The parents agree to encourage Haley to drink an additional three glasses of water per day, which they will often do together.

OUTCOME

After 3 months of regular meetings with the psychiatrist using principles of positive psychiatry, Haley and her family have made significant progress in many areas but lag in other areas. Overall, Haley's level of anxiety is much diminished, although her mother notes that "she's not exactly a social butterfly." The number of absences from school has dropped to about one per month. There remains some disagreements about how best to parent Haley, but both mother and father are now actively working together as a single unit.

Haley's mother made an appointment with her primary care physician regarding her own level of anxiety and is now taking sertraline with good results. The medication seems to be helping with her ability to follow through with some of the psychiatrist's recommendations for Haley, particularly those that involve some kind of exposure for Haley to participate in things that she is often reluctant to do at first. The father has declined a referral for a substance abuse evaluation but reports in the sessions with the psychiatrist that he has reduced his alcohol consumption and is actively trying to engage more positively with his wife and daughter. He has also been supportive of his wife's efforts to take care of herself, such as doing yoga twice a week.

Improvements have occurred in several areas of wellness and health promotion. The family is thrilled with the way that Haley has taken to the violin. She enjoys playing, practices, and has even agreed to participate in a recital in 2 months. Haley's enthusiasm for music has also inspired her mother to begin playing again on her own. The meditation sessions have also been well received, to the point that Haley herself will remind her parents to do them if they have forgotten. Hydration has improved, and Haley has successfully tried several new foods over the past few months.

Other areas of wellness, however, continue to be more of a challenge. The family did take two cross-country ski outings, which went relatively well, and in the warmer weather they regularly take walks after dinner. They admit, though, that getting Haley to be active every day is difficult without a lot of parental encouragement, and she continues to be quite unenthusiastic about joining a team. Their progress toward increasing Haley's giving back to others has also been slow. She was very uncomfortable in their sole attempt to return to church, and they have not returned. However, the mother recently learned of a charity 5K walk, and they have decided to do the walk together with another family.

With regard to sleeping, there have been some episodic evenings when Haley has been able to sleep in her room for the entire night, but these successes have not been consistent. The mother now feels more ready than she has in the past to prioritize Haley's sleeping habits, and the parents make a decision to begin the camping out technique in the evening.

In summary, Haley's family and psychiatrist are quite pleased with the progress made thus far and are encouraged by what appears to be a positive shift in developmental momentum. As is typical of this more wellness-oriented treatment, certain areas tend to gain traction for a family more readily than other areas, and therefore the clinician needs to continue to monitor progress or to adjust which domains receive the most focused attention. Haley's family agrees to continue working on their revised wellness plan and will continue to hold off on using any medications.

TAKE-HOME POINTS

- Positive psychiatry principles should now be considered evidence-based medicine and part of mainstream practice.

- A positive psychiatry approach opens a number of new avenues for intervention beyond individual psychotherapy and medications.

- Many clinicians can practice using a positive psychiatry approach without a major disruption in their practice habits.

- Like all treatments, a positive psychiatry–informed approach needs to be regularly reassessed and flexibly applied to fit the unique characteristics of each family.

REFERENCES

Achenbach TM, Rescorla LA: Manual for the ASEBA School-Age Forms and Profiles. Burlington, University of Vermont, Research Center for Children, Youth, and Families, 2001

Achenbach TM, Rescorla LA: Manual for the ASEBA Adult Forms and Profiles. Burlington, University of Vermont, Research Center for Children, Youth, and Families, 2003

Basoglu F, Rettew DC, Hudziak JJ: How much parental psychopathology is missed during standard child psychiatry evaluations? Poster presented at the annual meeting of the American Academy of Child and Adolescent Psychiatry, San Diego, CA, October 2014

Council on Communications and Media: Media use in school-age children and adolescents. Pediatrics 138(5):e20162592, 2016 27940794

Hudziak JJ: Genetic and environmental influences on wellness, resilience, and psychopathology: a family based approach for promotion, prevention, and intervention, in Developmental Psychopathology and Wellness: Genetic and Environmental Influences. Edited by Hudziak JJ. Washington, DC, American Psychiatric Publishing, 2008, pp 267–286

Hudziak J, Ivanova MY: The Vermont Family Based Approach: family based health promotion, illness prevention, and intervention. Child Adolesc Psychiatr Clin N Am 25(2):167–178, 2016 26980122

Ivanova M: Family Assessment and Feedback Intervention (FAFI): A Training Manual. Burlington, University of Vermont, Department of Psychiatry, 2013

Jeste DV, Palmer BW, Rettew DC, et al: Positive psychiatry: its time has come. J Clin Psychiatry 76(6):675–683, 2015 26132670

Kagan J: Galen's Prophecy. Boulder, CO, Westview Press, 1994

Lieb R, Wittchen HU, Höfler M, et al: Parental psychopathology, parenting styles, and the risk of social phobia in offspring: a prospective-longitudinal community study. Arch Gen Psychiatry 57(9):859–866, 2000 10986549

Patterson GR: Coercive Family Process. Eugene, OR, Castalia Press, 1982

Price AM, Wake M, Ukoumunne OC, et al: Five-year follow-up of harms and benefits of behavioral infant sleep intervention: randomized trial. Pediatrics 130(4):643–651, 2012 22966034

Rettew DC: Child Temperament: New Thinking About the Boundary Between Traits and Illness. New York, WW Norton, 2013

Rettew DC: Positive child psychiatry, in Positive Psychiatry: A Clinical Handbook. Edited by Jeste DV, Palmer BW. Washington, DC, American Psychiatric Publishing, 2015, pp 285–304

Schaefer JD, Caspi A, Belsky DW, et al: Enduring mental health: prevalence and prediction. J Abnorm Psychol 126(2):212–224, 2017 27929304

Siegenthaler E, Munder T, Egger M: Effect of preventive interventions in mentally ill parents on the mental health of the offspring: systematic review and meta-analysis. J Am Acad Child Adolesc Psychiatry 51(1):8.e8–17.e8, 2012, 22176935

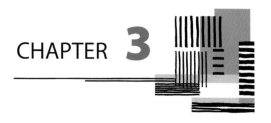

CHAPTER 3

A Strength-Based Approach to the Psychotherapeutic Management of Schizophrenia

Vihang N. Vahia, M.D., I.D.F.A.P.A.

Ambrish S. Dharmadhikari, D.P.M., D.N.B., M.A.P.A.

Editors' Introduction

This moving account of a woman with schizophrenia whose impressive recovery relies on positive interventions in the context of her Indian culture and supportive family brings up many important issues involved in the clinical application of positive principles. How much are these ideas embedded in particular cultures? What is the role of family in recovery and the positive psychiatry approach? How are traditional treatment modalities combined with positive interventions?

SUMMARY

Traditionally, clinicians associate the diagnosis of schizophrenia with poor prognosis. A history of psychotic symptoms that persist for over 3 years, coupled with a history of habitual nonadherence and subsequent poor response to conventional treatment, virtually clinches poor prognosis. The preferred treatment for schizophrenia continues to be drug therapy and psychoeducation aimed at rehabilitation and relapse prevention.

Mrs. M, a middle-aged woman diagnosed with paranoid schizophrenia and treated with drug therapy that helped partially, gave us newer insights into the thought process of a patient with schizophrenia. Her eventual return to premorbid functioning nearly 10 years after the onset of symptoms occurred when she could be gently persuaded to explore her own personal and professional competence. This strategy, coupled with helping the patient to accept the real-life adverse sequelae of her ailment and the possibility of leading an independent life, led to a commendable improvement in her quality of life as she regained her self-confidence and occupation.

PERSON

Mrs. M is a 45-year-old homemaker of Indian origin. Ten years before one of the authors (VNV) first examined her, she had migrated to New Zealand following her marriage. At the time of the examination, she had recently been released from a long-term mental health care facility in Auckland and deported to India for further management under her mother's care. She had been hospitalized in Auckland for aggressive and disruptive behavior. At the last admission, she had accused her husband of raping their daughter. She refused to accept that the news of her father's death was real. She accused the husband of being an imposter and insisted that she was married to Mr. Rahul Gandhi, a national political leader in India. She did not trust her husband and accused him of drugging her with potentially lethal medicines. She could not cope with day-to-day domestic chores of maintaining the house. She would neglect domestic tasks and other responsibilities, often challenging the family's right to expect her to manage the house simply because she was not employed. Her frequent episodes of aggressive outbursts had resulted in hospitalization in a long-term-care facility. Her mother, who visited the hospitalized daughter in Auckland, felt that she was incarcerated. During Mrs. M's last hospitalization in Auckland, her husband legally divorced her and the children disowned her.

Mrs. M, the younger of two sisters, was the product of a full-term normal delivery and was born to nonconsanguineous parents from upper socioeconomic strata. Her developmental milestones were normal. Her childhood was uneventful. Her mother described her as an impatient child with few friends. She was not willing to share her toys and belongings with others. Her mother remembers her as a good, well-behaved child so long as her few and otherwise acceptable demands were promptly fulfilled. Her schooling in a high-end private school and subsequent education up to a master's degree in commerce at Mumbai University were uneventful. She was reported to be a headstrong person who had few demands but who would not accept any alternatives to whatever she wanted. After completing her master's degree, she was employed in a chartered accountant's office, where she was assigned the task of keeping the books and filing income tax returns for clients. Her performance at work was reportedly rated as better than expected for a person of her level. After a year's experience at work, she willingly married her husband, whom she had never met, as arranged by her parents.

In her youth, she was given to mood swings, which were never considered as anything beyond the ordinary for an adolescent. Her father was fond of her, and she related better with her father. Her mother would at times feel that her father pampered her more than what was good for her. Her past and her family history were not contributory.

Mrs. M was unable to get suitable employment in New Zealand. She and her husband agreed that she could focus on managing her household chores and bringing up a family. However, she reportedly quarreled frequently with her husband. Her husband had complained to her parents that she was generally hostile and uncompromising. She compared her life after marriage unfavorably with her life as a single woman. Reportedly, her husband initially interpreted her episodes of aggressive behavior as a sign of her missing her parents, particularly her father. Over the years, her anger turned to hostile and assaultive behavior. She was reported to have accused her husband of poisoning her food after she questioned his fidelity. She had to be hospitalized for problems with controlling her aggressive behavior. She reprimanded her children because they were inclined to agree more often with her husband in the event of a quarrel in the house. She accused her children of conspiring with the father to prove her a lunatic. She habitually discontinued medication prescribed by the psychiatrists in Auckland. We were unable to obtain chronological data regarding the patient's hospitalizations or medical records from those hospital stays. Mrs. M's mother summarized her daughter's past medical history as multiple admissions lasting a few days to a few weeks, at the behest of her husband, to control her disruptive and aggressive outbursts. Her mother recalled that on a couple of occasions, police had to be called in to facilitate her daughter's hospitalization. Mrs. M was unable to provide any other data.

Seemingly, the episodes requiring hospitalization were of such severity that Mrs. M's husband was able to file for divorce on the evidence of her medical records. At the time of the divorce, the children opted to live with their father. The husband and the children continued to meet with Mrs. M often because she was staying in a separate part of the common house. Her husband and children, though legally divorced or separated, continued ensuring that her basic needs were met. They were prompt in seeking medical help for all her needs, including minor physical complaints. Eventually, she was admitted into a long-term mental health care facility, where she was treated with drug therapy and supportive care.

At this point, although her husband and children continued to pay for her health care and visit her at the hospital at regular intervals, specifically on occasions such as her birthday and culturally significant days, the family refused to consider having her return home. The remote possibility of her managing the family chores was clearly ruled out. She was given the choice of remaining in long-term care in New Zealand or returning to India to be looked after by her birth family. She insisted that she would remain in New Zealand so that she would be able to meet with her children and husband on whatever few occasions possible, although she did not like to meet her husband at all.

Six months before the present interview, after Mrs. M's father died, her mother concocted a story that her father was suffering from a serious illness. She did not reveal the news of his death to her daughter. Mrs. M's mother believed that she could trick her daughter into coming to India under the pretext of seeing her father. Mrs. M refused to believe that her father could be ill. Her mother counseled her about the possibility of living an independent life in India. The mother also assured her daughter that their relatives would be told that Mrs. M had opted to return to India because she was unhappy to be living away from her birth family and other relatives. Mrs. M was assured that the history of her mental illness would never be revealed to any of her friends and relatives. She was also cautioned that the offer to get her back to India was conditional on her agreeing to take regular medication.

In the interview with Mrs. M, just after she exhibited hypersalivation, stiffness, tremors, and anger against her mother and her sister, she complained of a pervasive sense of loneliness and betrayal. She said she was missing her children. Her mental status examination revealed that she was aware of the purpose of the psychiatric interview. She was cooperative and talked at length about her unhappy days in New Zealand. She was hostile and abusive against her sister and mother for getting her to return to Mumbai under the false pretext of her father being still alive and suffering from a potentially fatal illness. She said that in the past she used to hear some voices that made her do things but that those voices had not followed her when she returned to India. She expressed ideas of persecution. She accused her husband of conniving against her and of manipulating her mother and her sister to prove that she was seriously mentally ill. She had no insight. An observation considered to be of clinical significance was that at the very first interview Mrs. M thanked the interviewer (VNV) for being nonjudgmental. She appreciated that we had patiently listened to all that she had to say about her family in New Zealand and in India, without interrupting her narrative and without challenging her views. At the first interview, we seemed to establish rapport with Mrs. M, which was beneficial in all subsequent sessions. It was particularly noteworthy that she and her family had summarily refused the popular cultural view of faith healers and the views of the elders in her extended family that attributed her prolonged illness to celestial influences. Mrs. M and her mother had refused to accept alternative therapies.

FORMULATION

Mrs. M had presented with an indisputable diagnosis of paranoid schizophrenia. The course of the illness was adversely affected by her habitual nonadherence to treatment, which has been shown to lead to poor drug response. If the therapist and patient were to rely on drug therapy alone, without positive interventions to address, for example, nonadherence, the patient's illness would be labeled as refractory and in need of long-term drug therapy.

Surprisingly, at the first interview, at a time when she was being markedly aggressive and hostile toward her family and doctors, Mrs. M was able to form a rapport with us. This was an important observation, as well as a feature that could be woven into management strategy.

Positive psychology is in some ways an integral component of the joint family system in India. The treating primary care physician in India often assumes the traditional role of the "wise old grandparent who always knows what is good for every family member." This role of the family doctor is culturally acknowledged and usually accepted unchallenged. A family's doctors are consulted not only to have them examine and treat the sick and ailing in the family, but also to seek their advice on several other social and career-related issues. After all, every doctor is considered to be a highly educated and wise person who will do no harm to the patient. In Mrs. M's case, the treating psychiatrists' ages, ability to speak the patient's mother tongue, ability to converse about the nature of her work, nonjudgmental demeanor, encouragement of her efforts, and appreciation of her achievements further aided her recovery and rehabilitation.

INTERVENTIONS

The initial goal in the patient's management was to address any iatrogenic adverse drug effects. Mrs. M had agreed to take medicines as a precondition to her return to India; she agreed after learning that the dose could be tapered as appropriate. Clinically, she did not exhibit signs of gross personality deterioration, which would often be noticed in a case of chronic schizophrenia. This aspect of her clinical presentation was discussed with the patient and her mother. In this context, the family was informed of the clinician's decision to opt for positive psychological therapy in addition to continuing the oral antipsychotic drug therapy, aimed at rehabilitation and a return to Mrs. M's premorbid independent living. Mrs. M was informed of the importance of continuing the drug therapy. She was clearly told and she agreed that the shift from drug therapy alone to combined positive psychological therapy and drug therapy mandated her strict adherence to drug therapy.

The first step was to assess Mrs. M's strengths, weaknesses, opportunities, and threats—that is, to perform a SWOT analysis. The second step was to assess her degree of self-assurance and her optimism about leading a normal life. Both steps formed the foundation for her proposed therapy.

Step 1: Strengths, Weaknesses, Opportunities, and Threats (SWOT Analysis)

1. Strengths
   a. Mrs. M was a middle-aged intelligent person.
   b. She had strong family support. Despite being divorced, her husband continued to encourage her to lead an independent life. He volunteered to help her efforts.
   c. She was willing to take medicines.
   d. She was well educated. She had the potential to seek employment.
   e. She had the potential for generating revenue for her own independent living.
   f. Her hostility against her mother and sister was in some ways understandable and explainable.
   g. She was taking a low dose of an oral antipsychotic medication and was able to tolerate the drug well.

2. Weaknesses
   a. Mrs. M's illness had a long duration.
   b. She had a past history of habitual nonadherence to treatment.
   c. She wanted to return to New Zealand, even if she were to live away from her children and husband.
   d. She was reluctant to accept that regulatory authorities might not give her permission to return to New Zealand because she had been formally deported on grounds of mental illness that required constant care.
   e. She did not have any independent source of income.
   f. She was unable to form a lasting relationship or to make and sustain friends.

    g. Her husband and children were not willing to talk to her doctors in India or to any of her relatives other than her mother.

    h. It could not be confirmed whether the quality of support that Mrs. M mentioned was real or whether it was her wishful thinking.

3. Opportunities

    a. Mrs. M was a well-educated person who could be self-employed.

    b. Her cognitive functions were intact.

    c. Her close and extended family members in India were willing to help her to lead an independent life.

4. Threats

    a. Mrs. M had a history of nonadherence to treatment.

    b. It was not known how her husband would shape his life.

    c. Her emotional response if her husband ever remarried might cause a setback.

    d. She might have a setback if unable to attend important events in her children's lives, such as graduation and marriage.

    e. No information is available about the attitudes of her children and husband since her repatriation to India.

Step 2: Self-Assurance and Optimism

a. Mrs. M had a graduate degree in the field of commerce.

b. Her training could facilitate exploring an opportunity to work without having to deal with too many people, thus obviating any potential difficulties due to poor communication skills.

c. Her uncle, former colleagues, and clients were willing to help her find work.

d. Some of her previous clients were from her own family and religious fraternity groups.

e. The trustees of the temple where she had managed accounts in the past were willing to give her the responsibility of keeping the temple's books, albeit without remuneration.

f. Her family had already involved her in insurance and real estate sales jobs within their family's enterprise.

COURSE OF INTERVENTION

Mrs. M adhered to her single drug therapy of oral zuclopenthixol 10 mg/day, which was advised to her by her psychiatrists in Auckland. Zuclopenthixol is a typical antipsychotic drug belonging to the thioxanthene class. The drug can be administered orally or by intramuscular injections. It is a potent dopamine D_1 and D_2 receptor antagonist. It has high affinity for blocking α_1-adrenergic and serotonin 5-HT_2 receptors. This drug is favorably reviewed for its efficacy in management of acute disruptive episodes of psychosis and for maintenance treatment in the stable state of chronic positive symptoms of schizophrenia.

Mrs. M was willing to take prescribed medicines and requested management of her hypersalivation and tremors. Her blood tests revealed raised prolactin levels, dyslipidemia, and hypothyroidism. Two clinical considerations—oral zuclopenthixol is not available in India, and the patient was exhibiting extrapyramidal side effects from the drug—required that her medication be altered. She was thus switched to oral iloperidone 4 mg/day along with supportive benzhexol 2 mg twice daily, initially for a month before reassessment. One of the authors (VNV) told Mrs. M that daily morning and evening walks at her preferred time and pace would help. Her mother offered to accompany her on her walks, to which Mrs. M agreed.

Over the next 3 months following the initial interview, Mrs. M was found to be less hostile toward her mother and sister. She complained of boredom and said she was not occupied in any meaningful activities. Helping her mother and sister in cooking and housekeeping did not suit her. She said she was used to different styles of cooking, housekeeping, and managing domestic chores in Auckland. She said she could not adapt to the Indian pattern of managing the domestic chores. She insisted that her memory and her intelligence were not affected during her ordeal. She also mentioned a clear preference for a once-a-day medication.

Then, over the next 2 months, Mrs. M was remarkably well poised, talked about her hobbies, and stated that she indeed needed long-term medication. She was remorseful that during the previous 5 years she had been exhibiting such aggressive and disruptive behavior that her husband and children repeatedly had to take her to the hospital in Auckland. Every time, she would feel better with the prescribed medicines but would discontinue taking them because she did not see the need to continue them; adverse effects contributed to her nonadherence.

By this time in therapy, she was willing—in fact, wanting—to talk about her life since her marriage and her present state. She accepted that she had a long history of a major mental illness. She had read about her disorder on the Internet. She was aware that the disorder called schizophrenia is legally equated with insanity in that her civil rights are compromised. She was then made aware that nonadherence to treatment is the most common reason that a patient's schizophrenia might become chronic and potentially treatment resistant. Mrs. M was keen to return to Auckland, to be within easy reach of her children, and to rekindle her relations with her husband, who had not remarried. She was not willing to take "no" for an answer. We discussed the immigration laws of New Zealand, which mandate that a migrant have a steady and self-sustaining income. One of the authors (VNV) reminded her that in the previous year, she had been formally deported because of mental illness that required constant care. She then realized that she did not have any independent source of income. If she were to return to Auckland, she would be a burden on her children because she could not depend on her divorced husband to support her. She was aware that she was unable to bond with her friends and her family in Auckland. She said she found social interactions too monotonous and uninteresting. Activities like working out in a gymnasium or swimming where she could meet people and make friends did not appeal to her.

At this stage of her therapy, Mrs. M could be persuaded to consider exploring the prospects of engaging in a meaningful revenue-generating occupation. She said she had a degree in commerce and was proficient in bookkeeping. She had at some stage been helping a chartered accountant in Mumbai before she moved to Auckland after marriage. Some of the chartered accountant's clients used to outsource the task of maintaining accounts to her. She could recall names and contact details of some of her former clients.

She was receptive to the ideas of reviving her former business contacts and becoming engaged in revenue-generating and professionally meaningful activities. She opted to help an uncle who was an insurance agent. She was required to meet with potential clients and sell insurance policies. Because this job required communication skills and patience, it did not suit her well. She then opted to be a real estate agent; however, she felt that this profession was too strenuous and not rewarding.

After ruling out these jobs, Mrs. M recalled her training in accountancy, information technology, and computer-based accounting skills. She agreed to take a refresher course and familiarize herself with newer developments in that profession. She then acquired a personal computer and specialized accounting software to help her with maintaining customers' accounts. She was proud that she could acquire these materials from her own earnings over the past few months.

The mother was happy with her daughter's progress. She reported that Mrs. M was socializing with her relatives in India. She maintained cordial relations with her estranged husband and was quite caring of her children, whom she missed. In her work, she was able to deliver quality output and to cope with deadlines. She continued with her dose of iloperidone 4 mg/day. Her willful adherence to treatment decisively contributed to the remission of her clinical symptoms of suspiciousness, delusions, and aggressive behavior, and thereby facilitated recovery and socioeconomic-occupational rehabilitation.

As mentioned earlier, the intervention commenced with the realization that the personality of Mrs. M seemed well preserved and that she was willing to engage in conversations aimed at planning an independent future for her. The following theory construct, described in Step 3, began with the SWOT analysis discussed above.

Step 3: Positive Developments

a. Within a few weeks of agreeing to work in insurance sales and then as a real estate agent, Mrs. M earned small amounts of money.
b. This ability to earn money was a boost to her self-confidence.
c. The temple job was a boost to her social status and an indication that she could overcome the stigma of a broken marriage and deportation from New Zealand on grounds of her mental illness.

Step 4: Individualized Support System

a. Her mother, sister, and extended family in India supported Mrs. M.
b. The therapists ensured that Mrs. M appreciated the relevance of their attitude toward her and that she reciprocated the good gestures, such as their unconditional positive regard for her.

Step 5: Contributing Factors

a. Working for the family and the temple ensured that she was able to look beyond her family in Auckland.
b. She got into a structured routine of work and religious rituals, without feeling stigmatized.

Step 6: Looking Back Into Therapeutic Journey

a. When we look back, it is apparent that the examiner's noticing Mrs. M's demeanor at the first interview and her ability to be a part of a treatment regimen beyond drug administration set the path for her eventual return to her premorbid functioning.
b. She had received adequate drug therapy for her schizophrenia before the initial interview.
c. When Mrs. M was first examined, the positive aspects of her personality, personal life, intellectual strength, professional competence, family interactions, and state of illness were better appreciated.
d. Her clinical assessment at the time of the initial interview was a new beginning. The priority then was to address her iatrogenic symptoms.
e. It was soon apparent that she was willing to participate in therapy beyond drug taking.

f. The rapport she formed with the therapist facilitated an explanation of the aims of the therapy and prompted her to participate in redesigning her life. In more general terms, this rapport and its effect could be equated with the phenomenon of positive transference.
g. The therapist adhered to a strictly objective assessment and maintained professionalism, thus preventing any possibility of countertransference.
h. Mrs. M was adherent to the prescribed treatment.
i. She was regular with her work and her exercise routines.
j. She was willing to learn the updates of her profession.

OUTCOME

Mrs. M, a 45-year-old divorced woman diagnosed with schizophrenia of almost 10-year duration, was taking oral antipsychotic medication when we initially interviewed her. She had recently been deported from New Zealand to India. She had a history of short- and long-term hospitalizations in a mental health facility in New Zealand. She was habitually nonadherent to treatment.

After her involuntary return to India, she was able to establish good rapport with her psychiatrists. She adhered to the treatment that was planned for her. She was able to express her emotions and thoughts clearly to the psychiatrist. The focus of treatment shifted from symptom control to rehabilitation and return to premorbid level of functioning. Her family members in India, as well as her children and former husband abroad, were supportive of her. Family and well-wishers from the community helped her to regain her computer and accountancy skills. Her devotion to her religion and her contacts with the administrators of her temple facilitated her attempts to regain her self-confidence and obviate the stigma of being labeled as a mentally ill divorced woman.

Mrs. M has reconnected with her former business contacts and is now systematically increasing her workload. She continues to take oral iloperidone 4 mg/day. She follows a set exercise routine. Her social skills and interactions are better. She reports a significant improvement in her quality of life.

Her mother is pleased with her daughter's progress. The mother sometimes wonders whether her daughter ever suffered from schizophrenia or whether she was wrongly treated for a disease that she never had.

We are of the firm opinion that taking a "what-next" approach rather than indulging in the cause of all the patient's problems or finding faults with her husband and children helped Mrs. M to stop focusing on self-pity and instead explore means to restart her life. Mrs. M seems to be on the path toward satisfactory rehabilitation, while continuing to take a maintenance dose of an antipsychotic drug that is well tolerated and hence acceptable to her and her caregivers.

TAKE-HOME POINTS

- Positive psychological therapy addresses patient strengths and is particularly useful for patients who are not treatment compliant.

- Positive psychological therapy can enhance the therapeutic relationship and allow for improved collaboration involving psychopharmacological treatment.

- Family-centered approaches are consistent with positive psychological therapy.

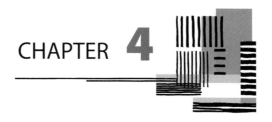

CHAPTER **4**

MDMA-Assisted Psychotherapy for Posttraumatic Stress Disorder

Andrew D. Penn, M.S., R.N., P.M.H.N.P.-B.C.

Marcela Ot'alora G., M.A., L.P.C.

Charles L. Raison, M.D.

Editors' Introduction

This extraordinary narrative of a woman with a trauma history who undergoes treatment with 3,4-methylenedioxymethamphetamine (MDMA) describes the transformation of her frightening and overwhelming inner memories and flashbacks into a powerful experience of safety and calm. The use of visual images and metaphor under the gentle guidance of the therapist, assisted by the pharmacological effect of MDMA, allows for a deeply moving and apparently persistent change in her subjective experience and identity.

The authors would like to acknowledge the subject of this case, SG, for her generosity and willingness to share her experiences in therapy. Additionally, we would like to acknowledge Sara Gael, M.A., and Saj Razvi, L.P.C., for their invaluable work with the patient.

SUMMARY

The patient (whom we will call SG) is a partnered woman in her late 30s with a lengthy history of posttraumatic stress disorder (PTSD). Specific details of her story have been changed to protect her identity. This case is being shared with her permission.

SG presented to the practice of one of us (AP) at the suggestion of a psychotherapist colleague who was working with her on Seeking Safety–based trauma skills (Najavits 2001) and exposure therapy for her chronic PTSD. The consultation question was whether medications might help SG's long-standing chronic PTSD.

SG had a history of sexual abuse from early childhood until early adolescence by a caregiver, with the abuse occurring in the context of willful neglect of this abuse from other caregivers. For approximately 20 years she has suffered from complex PTSD with prominent symptoms of hypervigilance, associated with feeling a lack of global sense of safety in her life.

PERSON

History

From as early as she could recall until approximately age 13, SG was subjected to ongoing sexual abuse from a caregiver. (SG has asked that the identity role of this person be withheld.) Additionally, another caregiver who had knowledge of this ongoing abuse at the time of its occurrence failed to act to prevent it from continuing, and at a later date, this caregiver attempted to discredit SG's claims of the abuse by questioning both the veracity of the claim and SG's mental health.

SG had been in individual interpersonal therapy for over 15 years and had recently completed a PTSD skills and exposure therapy group. She had tried complementary and alternative medicine treatments, including acupuncture and meditation, without significant benefit. She had been wary of using psychotropic medication, having only taken oxazepam for many years to address anxiety and sleep. She had never been psychiatrically hospitalized and, despite experiencing episodes of significant hopelessness, had never experienced suicidal ideation. She is a college graduate and works in the field of sales and marketing. She was previously married and was in a long-term relationship at the time of the intervention.

Diagnostic Assessment

The results of SG's ongoing and complex interpersonal childhood trauma were symptoms consistent with PTSD, including hypervigilance, avoidance of relationships with other people, intrusive memories, and constricted affect. Symptoms of major depressive disorder, anxiety disorders, psychotic disorders, personality disorders, and substance use disorders were absent.

SG showed symptoms of complex PTSD (not a DSM diagnosis), evidenced by her shame and her feelings of being damaged, unworthy of happiness or to have normal human relationships. van der Kolk (1996, 2014) and others describe complex PTSD as a change in multiple domains of psychological functioning as a result of trauma, particularly in alterations in self-perception, relationships with others, systems of meanings, and states of consciousness.

FORMULATION

Problems

SG exhibited classic DSM-5 symptoms of chronic PTSD, including hypervigilance, avoidance, intrusive memories, and constricted affect (American Psychiatric Association 2013). She described regular experiences of feeling horror, disgust, anger, sorrow, and shame when recalling her abuse experiences. These emotions often led to physical panic experiences of tachycardia, shortness of breath, and tremor.

Therapy became an aversive experience, and at times SG avoided it to prevent the exacerbation of intolerable PTSD symptoms. She described the "adult parts" of herself as able to understand cognitive restructurings of her trauma experience, but her "child parts," without a felt sense of safety, could not trust the therapist or the therapeutic process. Her defensive structures that permitted her to survive the abuse also prevented her from being able to feel vulnerable in therapy and therefore limited her ability to progress in treatment. This lack of progress in therapy added to a growing hopelessness that she would ever respond to treatment. Increasingly, she felt numb and removed not only from her experiences of the past but also from her ability to be present and feel a full range of emotions, including joy, in the present moment. She struggled with and found painful this inability to feel a full range of emotions. In her relationships, she felt self-loathing and unworthy of love.

Most concerning to SG was her growing hopelessness that she would ever recover from her experience and heal from her PTSD. Later, after completing the MDMA study, she admitted that she had been slowly losing hope and felt increasingly despairing that she would never improve.

Strengths

SG came to the MDMA-assisted psychotherapy trial with multiple strengths, the most significant being the absence of other significant psychopathology, personality disorder, or substance use disorders. She had a supportive long-term partner and had avoided the disruption of relationships often seen in people who survive long-standing childhood sexual abuse. She appeared to have excellent self-awareness, ability to tolerate emotional distress, and ability to self-regulate intense emotional states. She was also functional in her day-to-day life and had been able to maintain employment steadily through her adult life and, as a result, was able to provide for her own material needs. SG also came into treatment with superior verbal and written communication skills and a native intelligence for narrative therapy, which allowed her to express a largely ineffable experience of psychedelic experiences in the form of a complex but clearly meaningful narrative, described below (see "Interventions").

INTERVENTIONS

SG enrolled in the Colorado site of the Multidisciplinary Association for Psychedelic Studies (MAPS)–sponsored study of MDMA-assisted therapy for PTSD (Clinical Trials Registry No. NCT01793610), of which coauthor MOG is the principal investigator. In this Phase II pilot study, qualified patients were randomly assigned to receive preparatory psychotherapy with two study psychotherapists before receiving either 125 mg of MDMA, 100 mg of MDMA, or a 40-mg comparator dose of MDMA (a dose generally considered too low to have any therapeutic effect, therefore serving as an "active placebo") in a randomized, double-blind design. Subjects who remained within cardiovascular parameters following MDMA administration were offered a second "booster" dose 1.5 hours after the initial dose at a quantity of 50% of the first dose. This psychotherapy + MDMA intervention was repeated within 3–5 weeks of the first session at the same dose as in the first session. After the second session, the blind was broken and participants who received either 125 or 100 mg of MDMA were offered a third, open-label session with the same dose of MDMA used in the first and second sessions. Participants who received the 40-mg comparator dose were offered open-label treatment with a randomized dose of either 100 or 125 mg of MDMA with psychotherapy. SG was randomly assigned to the 125 mg of MDMA study arm and underwent three sessions at this dose, with the third session dose known to the patient and the study clinicians, per the open-label design.

The study's primary outcome measure was change in the Clinician-Administered PTSD Scale (CAPS) score, which was administered at baseline and 1 month after the second MDMA-assisted psychotherapy session. Additional outcome measures are described on the study's Web site (https://clinicaltrials.gov).

Why This Is a Positive Intervention

Positive psychiatry, with its emphasis on optimism, agency, autonomy, and hope, is well suited to help explain the psychotherapeutic benefits of MDMA-assisted psychotherapy for PTSD. This treatment for PTSD represents an extension of psychedelic-assisted psychotherapy models that were first pioneered in the 1950s in both Europe and North America by clinicians such as Stanislav Grof, Humphry Osmond, and Ronald Sandison, among others (Sessa 2013). As substances such as LSD (lysergic acid diethylamide) became diverted to the youth counterculture of the 1960s, a backlash resulted, leading to the Controlled Substances Act (CSA) of 1970, which was signed by President Richard Nixon. According to the CSA, Schedule I substances, including psychedelic compounds, are defined as having "no accepted medical use, a lack of acceptable safety for the use of the drug under medical supervision, and a high potential for abuse" (U.S. Food and Drug Administration 1970). This designation made conducting serious research on these substances impossible. When the National Institute of Mental Health–funded Maryland Research Center in Spring Grove, Maryland, ceased research on psilocybin in 1977, a period of nearly 30 years began during which no research was done on psychedelic-assisted psychotherapy in the United States (Richards 2016).

After this government-mandated interregnum, MDMA-assisted psychotherapy for PTSD began in 1996 with preliminary work published by Grob et al. (1996) and was followed up in 2000 with a study conducted by Michael and Annie Mithoefer in Charleston, South Carolina. Their work, published in 2011 (Mithoefer et al. 2011), showed that 83% of subjects treated with MDMA-assisted psychotherapy no longer had symptoms that met criteria for a PTSD diagnosis, compared with 25% of the subjects who received placebo treatment with psychotherapy. SG was a subject in an additional Phase II investigation into this treatment model, described in detail in the MAPS study treatment manual (Mithoefer 2013).

As with MDMA-assisted psychotherapy in general, the study in which SG participated administered MDMA for only a limited number of sessions. There was a total of 12 manualized psychotherapy sessions. MDMA was administered in only 3 of the 12 sessions.

Several putative neurobiological mechanisms have been identified by which MDMA may reduce PTSD symptoms following treatment. MDMA has been reported to attenuate amygdala responses to pictures of fearful or angry faces (Bedi et al. 2009) and/or reduce the connectivity between the amygdala and the left anterior temporal cortex when subjects are hearing their own narrative story of negative life events (Carhart-Harris et al. 2014).

This modulation of fear responses may facilitate the effectiveness of exposure therapy, which is a primary modality for the treatment of PTSD. Edna Foa (2011) describes exposure therapy, in which the person with PTSD is exposed to in vivo or in vitro cues of the trauma experience so that the anxiety response can be repeatedly elicited, eventually leading to an extinction of the pairing of cue and response. For this extinction to occur, the patient must be neither overwhelmed and flooded with the emotional response to the traumatic stimuli nor understimulated or disassociated by the exposure to the traumatic stimuli. The goal is an "optimum arousal zone," which allows the patient enough exposure to the feared stimuli to fully elicit the distress response, but not so much that the patient disengages or disassociates from exposure to the traumatic stimuli. It appears that MDMA, possibly via effects on the amygdala and related limbic structures, may help to reduce this neurological expression of fear and permit a freer exploration of traumatic memories that were previously aversive, with the result that patients reorganize a previously disorganized and distressing narrative into what has been called a "coherent narrative" of life events (Siegel 2015). If the narrative can change to become more coherent and less distressing, it is understandable how this might reduce the symptoms of PTSD.

Process of the Treatment: Sequence of Interventions and Assessment of Responses

Despite SG's wariness regarding the use of psychotropic medicines, she sought consultation in hopes of learning more about potential medication treatments for PTSD. We discussed, at length, standard treatments such as selective serotonin reuptake inhibitors and α- and β-noradrenergic antagonist medications. In response, she expressed apprehension about using daily medication. She asked if there were any new treatments being studied. She was informed about ongoing Phase II research on MDMA-assisted treatment of PTSD.

She was interested in knowing more and asked about the more common name of this drug. When we explained that MDMA is often called "ecstasy," she recalled a time in her early 20s when the memories of her childhood abuse were beginning to surface. At that time she had a boyfriend with whom she had taken ecstasy on several occasions (she stated that this was out of character for her, and she had not taken this or other psychedelic drugs since). When asked to recall what that experience was like for her, she replied, without hesitation, "It was the first time in my life I ever remember feeling safe. I see why it could be useful in therapy."

She asked if she could receive MDMA treatment from one of us (ADP) and was told that because it is a Schedule I drug, it could only be delivered in research settings. She asked for information about the trials and was provided with the Web site for ClinicalTrials.gov (https://clinicaltrials.gov) and the Web site of the sponsoring organization, MAPS (http://maps.org). On her own initiative, she then began to pursue enrollment in one of these trials, which was difficult because there was more demand than supply for this experimental treatment.

After 8 months, SG was enrolled as a subject in a Phase II trial with one of us (MOG) and the therapy team in Boulder, Colorado. This required her to make trips every 2–3 weeks over the next 3 months from California to Colorado.

Screening and assessment were completed using the CAPS, the Structured Clinical Interview for DSM-IV Axis I Disorders, Clinician Version (SCID-I; First et al. 1994), and the Structured Clinical Interview for DSM-IV Axis II Personality Disorders (SCID-II; First et al. 1997). SG's CAPS score at baseline was 108, indicating a significant burden of PTSD symptoms.

It is important to note that this treatment protocol is a psychotherapeutic one, enhanced by the use of MDMA as a catalyst to the healing process. MDMA serves to enhance the therapeutic process but is not therapeutic in isolation. Therefore, it is crucial to underscore the importance of the therapeutic relationship in psychedelic-assisted psychotherapy.

SG began meeting with her study therapists, a male-female dyad, who would work with her in preparing for the sessions, would sit with her for the duration of each session, and would do integrative psychotherapy in the days and weeks following the MDMA-assisted psychotherapy. She met with them three times, for 90 minutes each, before the first MDMA session to develop a therapeutic container, help them understand her history, and develop the expectations and trust needed to allow the therapeutic process to continue safely. As part of the preparation for the MDMA therapy sessions, there is intentional discussion about therapeutic use of touch during the session. Appropriate therapeutic, consensual, nonsexual touch, such as holding the hand of the therapist, can be a critical component of the therapy process. Many people with PTSD, especially those who have endured early childhood abuse, have not experienced healthy touch and can find the experience of appropriate physical contact to be therapeutic. Any physical contact between the patient and the therapist is always under the control of the patient, and any request to cease contact would be immediately honored. Additionally, the presence of a male-female dyad and the videotaping of all sessions provide additional security to both the patient and the therapists.

It is important to note that when compared with classical tryptamine psychedelic drugs such as LSD or psilocybin, the phenethylamine MDMA is typically less likely to cause visual hallucinations. Nonetheless, SG described her experience with MDMA-assisted psychotherapy as intensely narrative and richly symbolic, and it is that account which she shared with one of us

(ADP) in integrating the experience of the therapy at the completion of the clinical trial. At that time, she met with ADP for seven additional sessions to discuss and integrate her experiences in the study, which are described below. The phantasmagorical images she described can be seen as both a literal revisiting of events of childhood and a working-through of psychological themes expressed metaphorically.

MDMA SESSION 1

SG spent the night before her first MDMA-assisted psychotherapy session in a hotel. That night, while meditating on the upcoming events of the next day, she experienced a vision of herself as a fetus before birth, untouched by the abuse that she would experience in her childhood. She called this her "original self" and returned to this image repeatedly throughout the treatment sequence that followed over the succeeding 3 months.

The next morning, she reported to the study clinic. The therapy setting was a comfortable, living-room type of environment with a couch. Eyeshades and relaxing music via headphones were provided to reduce outside stimuli and allow her to direct her attention inward. She was given a capsule and then a booster 1.5 hours after the initial capsule. After the blind was broken, she and the researchers learned that the initial capsule and the booster contained 125 mg and 62.5 mg of MDMA, respectively. She reported that the first session commenced with some difficulty, as she experienced a sense of terror and became tremulous. She later realized that she was beginning to re-experience the felt sense of violation and fear that she had felt as a child. Usually a reserved person, she began to feel self-conscious about being vulnerable in front of the study therapists.

She experienced a vision of a massive black hole, a void, which came to represent the space and time in which her sexual abuse occurred. As a result of the psychedelic-induced perspective shifting, she was able to visualize herself as being inside the hole, looking up to the light and also looking down into the darkness within the hole.

Despite SG's self-conscious feeling of vulnerability in front of the therapists, the psychotherapy sessions she underwent before the MDMA session had provided her with a felt sense of nascent trust that allowed her to think that she might be able to heal herself through connection with other people. She recalled having the thought "I might be able to get out [from her past and her PTSD]," which she described as "the first deeply felt sense of hope I had experienced in my life."

As her perspective shifted, SG found herself sitting on the edge of this abyss, looking down into the hole. She saw a little girl, whom she would later recognize as a younger version of herself, approach her adult, first-person self. She watched the young child sit down next to her. The little girl suggested, "Why don't we look up at the sky?" SG described this experience as being "shown the way out…by my authentic self." This younger version of herself was to become a guide, a Virgil to her Dante, as she transited through the experiences occasioned in the MDMA-assisted psychotherapy.

Later in this first session, she saw a brilliant, bright blue light shining from the top of a pole and saw a suit of armor made of shining white metal. She felt that the light and the suit of armor represented both omniscience and "total protection," both of which were capable of keeping her out of harm's way as she proceeded through the next sessions.

Following the session, she wrote in her journal, "Your right to know what [safety] is like, to be in the world and not be cowering and to be safe. Believe in this. This is your right."

She later stated that after the first session ended, she had about 10 days with no symptoms of PTSD, and although this feeling faded after about 2 weeks, she was left with a residual knowledge that such a feeling was possible, and she told herself that it was important that she "[remember] this, so I don't forget," a kind of touchstone of possibility that she returned to frequently in the ensuing weeks of treatment.

BETWEEN MDMA SESSIONS 1 AND 2

Following the first MDMA session, SG stayed overnight at the clinic and was attended to by an overnight monitor. In the 3 weeks between the first and second sessions, she had several experiences of clinical importance. The first experience was a dream in which she was with the same little girl who had appeared at the edge of the abyss in the first session. As she and the girl were flying over a dark body of water that evoked, for her, the blackness of the abyss in the first session, she had the thought "I might be going in there [the dark water]," but she did not feel fear or apprehension.

Later, she spoke to her study psychotherapist about the parts of herself that she had to detach from as a child during her years of abuse. She was using the metaphor of shells that sea creatures discard, and that later wash up on the beach, as representing defenses of tender parts of her psyche that were wounded during the abuse. She realized that to defend herself, she had had to distance herself from normal parts of childhood, such as a sense of wonder or an intrinsic sense of being safe, and that she had felt alienated from those parts of herself for many years.

She also recalled that during the MDMA session, she experienced the felt sense that she had lived with while being abused as a child. She stated, "MDMA took me to the fear, the horror. It mirrored the same sense I had as a child, the same fear and horror. [MDMA] was not warm and fun."

At a later session with the study therapist during which she was discussing how trauma treatment challenges the long-standing defenses she had held since childhood, she had a daydream of a piñata surrounded by younger it-erations of herself at ages 2, 6, and 9 years, and imagined the study therapist tossing her a stick that she used to break open the piñata, which contained what she described as "insights."

In another psychotherapy session, she was exploring how as a child she had to believe the distortions of her abuser because she was dependent on that person. She discussed how later in life, when she began to tell others about the abuse she suffered as a child, the abuser raised questions of her credibility by saying that she was severely mentally ill. She thought, "What if I don't believe their lies anymore?" and felt that she had begun the process of "liberating myself from the abuser's story."

MDMA SESSION 2

SG reported that she went into the second MDMA-assisted psychotherapy session (again, a blinded dose that was later revealed to be 125 mg followed by a 62.5-mg booster dose 1.5 hours later) with a sense of apprehension and doubt, thinking, "I'm crazy, I'm wasting their time." This feeling of dysphoria and anxiety persisted as the drug began to take effect. She felt regressed to being 5 years old and felt as if she were hiding under the bedsheets. She stated that she felt physically uncomfortable, wanting to get off the study couch and to take off the eyeshades that were used to screen out unnecessary visual stimuli. She felt a certain degree of fear of the study therapists, which she later realized was part of her historical PTSD response but unwarranted by the current circumstances. She wanted to leave the room but knew this was not allowed under the study protocol. She had considerable apprehension about taking the booster dose of MDMA at 1.5 hours. She realized that if she took the optional dose, there was "no going back."

SG began to reframe her abuse in her mind as something she had survived, and to realize that she was making a conscious choice to return to recalling the trauma. She remarked, "It was like walking back into hell. I would see my younger self, who would run away from me saying, 'I don't trust you. You [adult self] left me here in this hell. You never listened to me; you left me here in this house.'" She decided to take the second dose as a way of inten-tionally choosing to go back into the trauma memories. She later remarked, "I've had to become an amazing parent to myself. My fear, my anxiety, my in-somnia made sense, became perfectly congruent…. In trauma, nothing feels safe. You don't know why you feel anxious. I was getting all my parts back."

Later in the second MDMA session, SG imagined herself back in the house of her childhood where her abuse took place. She found an old key that she intuitively knew "unlocked" the past story. She described the experience as retuning to and reexperiencing her childhood home and engaging with the younger version of herself that was locked in the house as she was being abused. She felt compelled to free her from the house, but said that when she found the young child version of herself, the child was wary and did not trust her.

Regaining the trust of this "inner child" who had experienced abandonment in the midst of the abuse became a critical theme of the second MDMA session. Despite the fear that she experienced earlier in the session, SG stated that she made a conscious decision, which she expressed to one of the therapists, that she wanted to keep going more deeply into her trauma material.

She felt that she could transfer the wisdom and knowledge that she had gained about her abuse and about trauma to the younger version of herself, and by doing so, she hoped she would feel connected to that younger part of herself. A scene occurred in which the adult and child parts of herself reconciled, and the younger version of herself was able to give voice to feeling abandoned and left in a harmful environment. In response, the adult version of herself was able to acknowledge the pain that this abandonment had caused her. She described that she and her younger child self felt liberated and joyful after this reconciliation.

From this point onward, the younger version of herself became a frequent companion to the first-person adult during the MDMA sessions. This was not a psychotic or dissociative phenomenon, because SG was well aware that this person represented a younger version of herself from whom she had become estranged during her abuse and in later years. The reconciliation between this younger, wounded part of herself and her current adult self was to become a recurring and important theme in the therapy.

After this reconciliation, SG found herself with her younger self in a variant of her childhood bedroom, except there were no doors. She was holding a mirror that reflected an image of the people who had abused her. She realized in that moment that she was not going to get an apology from them, and that she now had the courage to look at the truth of what had occurred when she was a child.

She then saw her younger self in a scene of sexual abuse. She remembered feeling the physical sensation of being violated. She recalled a sense of disaffection, thinking how routine the abuse had become, but also recalled thinking as a child, "This is all I'm good for." But in the MDMA psychotherapy session, she questioned that assumption and had the spontaneous thought that "I know I'm worth more."

The second MDMA session came to a close, and again SG stayed at the clinic with an overnight safety monitor. As she was getting ready for bed, she had a spontaneous memory of being about 8 years old and contemplating committing suicide in a violent and gory manner to communicate to her abusers how much pain she was in, and how enraged she was at being abused. The next morning, she went on a hike; thinking about the choice not to end her life as a child, she felt gratitude that she had lived, and she honored the younger part of herself that chose not to act on the suicidal impulse that she had felt many years before.

BETWEEN MDMA SESSIONS 2 AND 3

Between the second and third sessions, SG recalled a dream in which she was inside an empty sea cave when a massive wave entered the cave and battered her against the stone in darkness. She awoke thinking, "What has this therapy done to me? Maybe the enormity of this is too much for me." She discussed this with one of the study therapists, who reassured her that she would be okay. She found this reassurance to be very powerful, stating, "She had faith in me, even when I didn't have it in myself."

Additionally, in the therapy sessions between MDMA sessions 2 and 3, SG began to develop a greater sense of trust in her own recollection of events from childhood, something that had always been difficult for her after her veracity had been questioned in the past.

She discussed how the therapy sessions helped her to integrate her feelings about her life at a younger age with how she saw her life now. She experienced grief at the memory of what she now considered "self-betrayal"—for example, when she used alcohol (in the past) and anxiolytic medication to avoid "all the things I couldn't handle or address." She stated that when she was younger, she felt that "when I left home, I was never going home again, but with MDMA [therapy], I went home again. I wish I could have done this when I was younger, before I had amassed negative experiences, failures, and negative self-beliefs."

MDMA SESSION 3

SG arrived at the third session with confidence, stating, "I arrived as my adult self. Something amazing happened. I knew how to do the work of healing. I grew. I was present as an adult for the first time, and I was ready. The little girl was ready to go with me. We went in as a team, and I didn't know what to expect, but I knew I could handle it." She went on to say that she expected to encounter traumatic material again, as she had in the first two sessions, but that this time "the old demons aren't truth anymore. I had to go in to tear them down."

For this session, SG received an open-label dose of 125 mg of MDMA without the 50% booster dose because of transient hypertension, above the study cutoff, that occurred after receipt of the initial dose. As the MDMA began to take effect, she set an intention to connect with the most wounded parts of herself. She envisioned a beautiful light and found herself drawn to it. She also knew that she needed to work with darker parts of her experience, but she realized that doing that would not diminish the metaphorical experience of light and that, in fact, the younger parts of her were an embodiment of this light.

At this point, she had a transference-type experience with the male study therapist, asking him, "Can you look at me as if I were your child, so that I know that I am cherished?" He said he could do this, and she found this experience to be healing and corrective, as she felt that she could both be cherished and have her boundaries respected. She reported, "I asked the therapists for human connection, to be held." She reported that the safe, consistent, and appropriate physical contact with the therapists allowed for the development of significant trust, which facilitated deeper exploration of her trauma.

Going forward in the session, she made a conscious decision to go back into the trauma material, and again she encountered her inner younger self, who told her, "I'm ready to take you," at which point she found herself descending into the earth in a cage. She described this as being "like I was going thousands of feet [down] within myself." She instructed the younger part of herself to stay "aboveground" where she would be safe.

When this descent stopped, she found herself alone, outside a massive cage, some 40 feet tall, with bars as thick as trees. She noticed an opening between the bars and decided to enter. It was very dark inside. Inside the cage, she saw spheres, like cannonballs, arranged in circles on the ground. Once she was in the middle of the cage, multiple images of her abuser arose from the spheres like holograms. He was naked and omnipresent. She felt surrounded and trapped. She quickly left the cage, feeling terrified.

She opened her eyes and told one of the therapists what she had seen. The therapist asked her, "What can you bring into the cage?" She recalled the light that she'd evoked in meditation at the start of the session and decided to bring it into the cage. She said, "Okay, I'm going back in there. I'm going to bring this radiant light back in there. It's not so scary. I have light, power, and truth. I'm out of the shadows."

She reentered the cage, this time bearing a bright light, and again saw the figure of her abuser inside the cage. This time, the multiplicity of images of him had been replaced with only one figure, and he was naked, afraid, and ashamed, running away from her to the dark corner of the cage, away into the darkness. She thought, "I see you for who you are." She later described in an integrative psychotherapy session the thought that "the shame I have been carrying my whole life is not my shame. It's his shame, and I don't have to carry it anymore." She credited MDMA with her ability to tolerate the shame that she usually felt when thinking about her abuse and to have more options with which to interpret the experiences of her childhood.

With the abuser figure now gone, she lifted up one of the spheres that littered the floor of the cage. Although it was heavy, she was able to throw it on the ground, where it cracked into two perfect hemispheres. She described the interior of one of the spheres as having a bucolic scene of a meadow full of flowers. The other half contained a violent memory of her childhood abuse, with all the attendant emotions of pain, fear, and horror. She felt like she had a choice about where to direct her attention. She felt like she had the courage, because of the MDMA, to enter the scene of abuse and to comfort her younger self and reassure her that she would be okay. She then experienced a compassionate distance from the experience and the suffering she experienced.

After this scene, she found herself descending through the earth again, with the younger part of herself having rejoined her at her side. She emerged in a large, ornate, gilded ballroom that was brightly lit and beautiful. She and the younger part of herself twirled, back to back, around the dance floor. She described feeling a sense of wonder and awe at the spaciousness and the decor. She noticed that there were spheres, similar to those in the cage, on the floor, but they were not just black; there were both colorful spheres and black spheres. She realized that the spheres represented different memories in her life, and although the black memories (of trauma) still existed, they were now contextualized in the whole of her life. In an integration psychotherapy session, she later remarked, "More memories will surface, and that will be okay."

Later, after the MDMA session was complete and she was contemplating these images, SG began to think about suffering, and about her self-identity as a damaged, unwanted, uncared-for survivor of sexual abuse. She summarized this reframing of her experience by saying, "These things happened to me, but they are not who I am." She began to realize that for the first time in her life, she could assume that her current life had a reasonable margin of safety rather than assume the world was always dangerous.

SG discussed with one of us (ADP) how the treatment had changed her symptoms of PTSD. She discussed her lifelong recurrent nightmares of being hurt in bed, where most of the abuse had occurred. She stated, "Lifelong insomnia was the most debilitating part of my PTSD, but I'm not afraid to go to sleep now." SG also discussed how she left the treatment study with a changed outlook, characterized by a deeply embodied sense of hope. She remarked, "It's not something you talk about. It's something you feel."

Therapeutic Relationship

The relationship between therapist and client is unique in MDMA-assisted psychotherapy. In the case of SG, the experiences occasioned by MDMA provided safety and trust in the self early on in the treatment. In general, as clients experience themselves less defensively and with greater acceptance, their sense of wholeness emerges and genuine connection is possible. When an authentic self emerges, there is room for truth and compassion for all parts of the self, creating fertile ground for healing to take place.

The therapist's responsibility in the alliance is to be authentically present without the need to "do" something. A mindset that has been characterized as "beginner's mind" (Suzuki 1970) is an essential component, because it allows for curiosity and a nonjudgmental stance that brings spaciousness and safety to the container being developed. The therapist's role is not to "give" something to the client but to be engaged in the act of empathic attunement. Empathy grows out of the desire to fully understand the client and becomes a potential antidote to the shame clients often feel and are weighed down by. As a witness, the therapist is affected by the client's experience and also feels his or her own self-empathy.

Interweaving of Traditional Psychiatric Interventions With Positive Interventions

Traditional psychotherapeutic approaches to help patients afflicted by trauma seek to reduce their maladaptive responses to internal and external trauma cues (e.g., hypervigilance, avoidance, withdrawal) and to return patients to a kind of autonomic homeostasis when presented with reminders of the trauma. One example of this type of approach is prolonged exposure, an evidence-based behavioral therapy that seeks to overcome avoidance of trauma cues, which is common for patients with PTSD, by repeated and controlled exposure to memories and reminders of the traumatic event(s). Eye movement desensitization and reprocessing (EMDR) derives from a similar therapeutic model and adds bilateral stimulation of the brain through alternating, lateralized visual, auditory, or tactile stimuli that are used while the patient is recalling traumatic memories. Although effective, both therapies are often difficult for patients to tolerate, and the dropout rate is high. It is clear that although both of these modalities have contributed greatly to the treatment of PTSD, additional, more tolerable methods are needed.

MDMA-assisted psychotherapy utilizes an eclectic methodology (Mitheofer 2013) that includes aspects of exposure therapy, internal family systems therapy, cognitive-behavioral therapy, narrative therapy, Holotropic Breathwork (a means of generating and working with non-drug-induced nonordinary states of consciousness developed by Grof and Grof (2010), and somatic-based therapy modalities such as Somatic Experiencing (Levine 2010) and Hakomi therapy (a mindfulness-based, somatically organized psychotherapy model) (Kurtz 2007). Because the therapy involves far more than merely administering the drug, it is clear that the therapeutic relationship established at the onset, continued through the MDMA psychotherapy sessions, and enduring through the integration of the treatment, is a critical aspect of the psychotherapy.

An important premise of MDMA-assisted psychotherapy is that the client is the expert and already holds the capacity needed for healing and the healing takes place not by getting rid of something, but rather by making room for the inner, innate healing intelligence to emerge. Therapists bring into the room their own resources and preferred therapeutic modalities but hold these lightly, suspending agendas and remaining conscious that their interventions are in the service of supporting awareness and must not impede the patient's present-moment experience.

Therapeutic skills are used to clarify when there is confusion or the client is stuck and to solidify integration. Therapeutic theories complement the process of the patient but are not the centerpiece of the work. MDMA provides a grounding field in which the client is able to experience a sense of connection between mind, body, and spirit in the present moment, which allows for integration to take place through the senses in a nonlinear manner. The therapist's role is to follow and to be a witness to the unfolding process.

Therapeutic modalities that support this process are those that focus on the body as an agent of truth since the body becomes the guide and informs movement. Therapies that work with transpersonal experiences as a way of understanding connection to self and other are also useful. MDMA facilitates experiences in which the client can hold several perspectives at the same time and can often experience the self and the observer simultaneously.

Therapies, such as internal family systems (Schwartz 1997), that focus on bringing awareness to "parts" of the self are helpful, given that marginalized aspects of the self emerge naturally during MDMA therapy. When this occurs, the experience typically promotes a sense of permission from protective parts of the self to explore wounded parts that have previously not been given a voice. This capacity for integrating representations of oneself from an earlier age was also noted in a qualitative study of participants in a psilocybin-assisted psychotherapy protocol for patients with life-threatening illnesses (Belser et al. 2017).

Attachment themes often emerge. With a male-female dual-therapist model, the therapists hold different transferential roles during the session and are often secure attachment figures available to the patient for contact and bonding. Consistent with this, the working-through of transferential material appears to have been a critical part of the improvement experienced by SG as a result of the treatment.

In their seminal article on positive psychology, Seligman and Csikszentmihalyi (2000) emphasize the importance to positive psychology of realistic, even stoic, optimism, based in autonomy and self-determination. As SG transited through her treatment, her optimism grew from a vague hope that things could improve to a confidence that despite her past trauma she would be able to live a fulfilling life. Because of this, her healing came not from forgetting the trauma she had experienced, but rather from learning to maintain a dispassionate yet self-compassionate stance toward her own experience. She states that she now has a different relationship with trauma-related symptoms, such as anxiety, and is more able to sit with the distress created by the emotion, and feels less compelled to run from the feeling. She stated in a later interview, "I have happiness. I have love. I also have anxiety. It's just okay. I listen to all of me."

Posttraumatic growth, defined as wisdom and meaning emerging out of traumatic experiences, has been discussed extensively among advocates of positive psychology (Calhoun and Tedeschi 1998) and existential psychotherapy (Frankl 1946). Such growth emphasizes changing the valence of a traumatic event from one of victimization without agency toward one of perspective and growth despite adversity. Certainly, the perspective that SG gained through her MDMA-assisted psychotherapy is an example of such growth. Ongoing Phase II MDMA-assisted PTSD therapy studies are using the Posttraumatic Growth Inventory as a secondary outcome measure (Mitheofer 2013).

OUTCOME

How the Treatment Ended

SG's experimental treatment ended after completion of the integration sessions that followed the third MDMA psychotherapy study session. Psychometric measurements were completed at the end of the treatment. Her CAPS score had dropped from 108 prior to treatment to 51 at the end of the study. A CAPS score of ≥50 indicates moderate to severe PTSD, and a drop of ≥ 30% is considered a clinical response (Mithoefer et al. 2011).

SG returned from Colorado and resumed psychotherapy with one of us (ADP) in California. She reported feeling significantly better and deeply grateful for the treatment. She and ADP discussed what she felt she needed going forward. She asked for additional opportunities to discuss her experiences and process the MDMA treatment sessions and integration. She and ADP met for about 12 hours over the course of seven sessions. She stated that she wished she could draw some of the images she had seen during the MDMA sessions but that her artistic skills were limited. One of the study staff suggested she use Google Image Search to find approximations of what she saw during the therapy sessions. She used the images she found to make approximately 75 storyboard cards that she used in integrating the sessions. She stated that the process of making the cards helped her to organize her experiences and to create a cohesive narrative of her story, which was additionally therapeutic.

Symptoms and Positive Experiences, Strengths, and Satisfaction

A year after the treatment, SG continued to be clinically free of PTSD. Her CAPS score continued to drop in that ensuing year, from 51 at study endpoint to 26 at 1-year follow-up. She continued to use hypnotic medication about 5–8 nights per month but takes no other psychotropic medications. She has not used MDMA again and has no interest in using it outside a therapeutic environment. In later interviews, she described the MDMA psychotherapy process as a kind of "inverted PTSD" in that by reversing the slow accretion of childhood trauma that led to the burden of PTSD symptoms, this therapy slowly allowed her to increase her feelings of safety and thereby unburdened her from the symptoms of PTSD.

She has been able to make changes in her work and personal relationships that required her to make some difficult decisions. She feels that she has been able to end relationships that were no longer working for her and to act more decisively in her own best interests. She reports, "I often feel a deep, heartfelt sense of joy for simply being alive and fully present in the moment." She has been more able to utilize therapy and meditation to further advance her healing. She reports feeling more connected with the important people in her life.

She is deeply appreciative of having been included in the study. Because of the high media profile of the experimental treatment, she has been approached to speak about her experiences publicly at conferences or in media interviews. She has thus far declined these invitations, but she has permitted us to share her story in professional and educational settings, because she feels it is important that the community of mental health clinicians know about the potential benefits of this treatment protocol.

Assessment of the Patient's Progress and Response

In our clinical opinion, SG has markedly improved as a result of her MDMA-assisted psychotherapy treatment. Her symptoms of PTSD remain largely absent. Her use of psychotropic medication is minimal. She has improved her functioning in both interpersonal and occupational spheres. She told about asking for a raise at work, recalling the time in the treatment where she realized she was worth much more than just being the victim of abuse; this realization had bolstered her confidence. These gains have persisted for more than 1 year after her last MDMA-assisted psychotherapy session.

Why the Positive Intervention Mattered

The experience of long-standing trauma, especially early in life, not only creates the symptom cluster of hypervigilance, avoidance, reexperiencing, and mood disruption that is categorized as PTSD, but also often deeply damages the sense of self and the narrative of how one came to be an adult. The experience of trauma becomes central to the sense of self. Qualities deeply valued by positive psychology, such as optimism and autonomy, are often profoundly impacted. The clinically supervised and time-limited use of MDMA that occurs within a psychotherapeutic relationship may allow for a rewriting of the trauma narrative through the eyes of the adult in a way that promotes a deeply held sense of mastery over one's experience. Trauma memories, no longer central, can now share space with experiences of the current, adult self. The enhancement that MDMA provides to the psychotherapeutic relationship has the potential to allow for a felt sense of trust. For SG, MDMA-assisted psychotherapy allowed her to have for the first time a deeply felt experience of safety, upon which she was able to build a foundation for additional healing and growth.

TAKE-HOME POINTS

- Studies to date suggest that 3,4-methylenedioxymethamphetamine (MDMA)–assisted psychotherapy is a safe and effective treatment modality for posttraumatic stress disorder (PTSD).

- MDMA-assisted psychotherapy for PTSD allows those who have experienced trauma to explore their experience in a safe therapeutic setting.

- Posttraumatic growth, a key concept in positive psychology, is a likely outcome of MDMA-assisted psychotherapy for PTSD.

- The cautious and controlled use of MDMA-assisted psychotherapy for PTSD may allow people who have experienced trauma to revise their narrative of the traumatic experience in a way that renders them in control of their experience, rather than as the victim of circumstance.

REFERENCES

American Psychiatric Association: Diagnostic and Statistical Manual of Mental Disorders, 5th Edition. Arlington, VA, American Psychiatric Association, 2013
Bedi G, Phan KL, Angstadt M, et al: Effects of MDMA on sociability and neural response to social threat and social reward. Psychopharmacology (Berl) 207(1):73–83, 2009 19680634
Belser AB, Agin-Liebes G, Swift TC, et al: Patient experiences of psilocybin-assisted psychotherapy: an interpretive phenomenological analysis. Journal of Humanistic Psychology 57(4):1–35, 2017

Calhoun LG, Tedeschi RG: Beyond recovery from trauma: implications for clinical practice and research. J Soc Issues 54:357–371, 1998

Carhart-Harris RL, Wall MB, Erritzoe D, et al: The effect of acutely administered MDMA on subjective and BOLD-fMRI responses to favourite and worst autobiographical memories. Int J Neuropsychopharmacol 17(4):527–540, 2014 24345398

First MB, Spitzer RL, Gibbon M, Williams JBW: Structured Clinical Interview for DSM-IV Axis I Disorders (SCID-I), Patient Edition (SCID I/P). Washington, DC, American Psychiatric Press, 1994

First MB, Spitzer RL, Gibbon M, et al: Structured Clinical Interview for DSM-IV Axis II Personality Disorders (SCID-II), Washington, DC, American Psychiatric Press, 1997

Foa EB: Prolonged exposure therapy: past, present, and future. Depress Anxiety 28(12):1043–1047, 2011 22134957

Frankl VE: Man's Search for Meaning. Boston, MA, Beacon Press, 1946

Grob CS, Poland RE, Chang L, et al: Psychobiologic effects of 3,4-methylenedioxy-methamphetamine in humans: methodological considerations and preliminary observations. Behav Brain Res 73(1–2):103–107, 1996 8788485

Grof S, Grof C: Holotropic Breathwork: A New Approach to Self-Exploration and Therapy. Albany, State University of New York Press, 2010

Kurtz R: Body Centered Psychotherapy: The Hakomi Method. Mendocino, CA, Life-Rhythm Books, 2007

Levine PA: In an Unspoken Voice: How the Body Releases Trauma and Restores Goodness. Berkeley, CA, North Atlantic Books, 2010

Mithoefer MC: A manual for MDMA-assisted psychotherapy in the treatment of posttraumatic stress disorder. Multidisciplinary Association for Psychedelic Studies, January 4, 2013. Available at: http://www.maps.org/research-archive/mdma/MDMA-Assisted_Psychotherapy_Treatment_Manual_Version_6_FINAL.pdf. Accessed November 11, 2017.

Mithoefer MC, Wagner MT, Mithoefer AT, et al: The safety and efficacy of ±3,4-methylenedioxymethamphetamine-assisted psychotherapy in subjects with chronic, treatment-resistant posttraumatic stress disorder: the first randomized controlled pilot study. J Psychopharmacol 25(4):439–452, 2011 20643699

Najavits LM: Seeking Safety: A Treatment Manual for PTSD and Substance Abuse. New York, Guilford, 2001

Richards W: Sacred Knowledge: Psychedelics and Religious Experience. New York, Colombia University Press, 2016

Schwartz R: Internal Family Systems Therapy. New York, Guilford, 1997

Seligman ME, Csikszentmihalyi M: Positive psychology: an introduction. Am Psychol 55(1):5–14, 2000 11392865

Sessa B: The Psychedelic Renaissance: Reassessing the Role of Psychedelic Drugs in 21st Century Psychiatry and Society. London, Muswell Hill Press, 2013

Siegel D: The Developing Mind: How Relationships and the Brain Interact to Shape Who We Are, 2nd Edition. New York, Guilford, 2015

Suzuki S: Zen Mind, Beginner's Mind. New York, Weatherhill Press, 1970

U.S. Food and Drug Administration: Controlled Substances Act. 1970. Available at: https://www.fda.gov/regulatoryinformation/lawsenforcedbyfda/ucm148726.htm. Accessed November 13, 2017.

van der Kolk BA: The body keeps the score: memory and the evolving psychobiology of posttraumatic stress disorder, in Traumatic Stress: The Effects of Overwhelming Experience on Mind, Body, and Society. Edited by van der Kolk BA, McFarlane AC, Weisaeth L. New York, Guilford, 1996, pp 214–241

van der Kolk BA: The Body Keeps the Score: Brain, Mind, and Body in the Healing of Trauma. New York, Viking, 2014

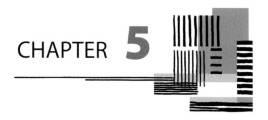

CHAPTER 5

Recovering Strengths

Combining Psychodynamic Psychotherapy and Positive Psychiatry for Improved Self-Esteem

Behdad Bozorgnia, M.D., M.A.P.P.

Editors' Introduction

The integrated psychodynamic and positive psychotherapy described in this chapter demonstrates the synergy of the two approaches and also some of the technical challenges. The positive psychiatrist modified the traditional positive approaches to fit the patient's core psychodynamic problem so as to enhance their effectiveness and not play into resistances. The case study demonstrates how empathy in the therapeutic relationship helps the patient enhance his or her ability to experience positive emotions.

SUMMARY

John, a 17-year-old college student majoring in computer engineering and economics, has a past history of social anxiety and presents with worsening anxiety and depression in the setting of starting a heavy course load during the first semester of his freshman year. His early childhood experiences of unpredictable and intense parental rage led him to fear his own emotions and struggle with expressing anger and aggression. His fear led to a deep self-consciousness and an avoidance in social situations. The patient also had, accompanying and underpinning his social anxiety, difficulty regulating his self-esteem, often oscillating between the poles of superiority and inferiority in relation to his peers. His dichotomous self-image led to a pattern of constantly comparing himself to others, which further undermined his ability to form close and meaningful relationships. The therapy was mainly psychodynamic and consisted of both expressive techniques to uncover the repressed aggressive affect behind this young man's anxiety and supportive techniques to repair his sense of a damaged self. The psychological process of healing was concomitant with the positive processes of developing the capacity to love and be loved as well as the strength to be forgiving, especially of himself.

Person

When I first met John, it was early autumn and the leaves were just starting to lose their summer luster. We met once a week at a college counseling center for 1-hour therapy sessions involving mostly supportive and expressive techniques. The first time he walked into my office, I was struck by how his fashionable and casually preppy style of dress contrasted with his shaggy but still cropped jet-black hair. He was very polite; he thanked me when I held the door for him and often expressed gratitude as each session came to a close. After several weeks he sat low and comfortable in a consulting chair in an almost devil-may-care posture. He engaged in eye contact only intermittently and spent the majority of the time looking down at the corner of the room. He talked in an informal yet somewhat distant tone, often interspersed with bursts of self-directed laughter.

He initially complained of constantly worrying about what other people thought. Specifically, he felt anxious that others would judge him harshly in class or at parties, thinking that he was stupid, awkward, and undoubtedly uncool. His anxiety was so intense that it often prevented him from raising his hand in class when he had an idea to share. Instead of participating, he ruminated on how his ideas and thus his character would be judged as stupid or unworthy. He avoided social gatherings for fear of seeming awkward or socially inept. He spent hours thinking about how others would think that he was not smart enough and that he was somehow odd or defective. He had friends but did not consider any of them particularly close or intimate. Although he was very gifted and generally doing well in his classes, he often avoided or showed up late to small groups.

John had recently moved from a small town to a large metropolis to start college at a prestigious and competitive university, where he was majoring in both computer science and engineering. He also worked a campus job and was actively engaged in several clubs. He took a large course load and spent much of his time on his classwork. At times, he stayed up until the early hours of the morning working on his assignments. His schedule was a tight bundle of activities, which seemed timed to the minute. He was teeming with an almost compulsive ambition that led him to work with such drive that he showed little consideration for his own self-care. His schedule was packed with classes, activities, and meetings, and his sleep, nutrition, and exercise habits often took a backseat to these. He wanted not only to do well in his course work but to be "the best." We had many conversations about the ultimate distinction between GPAs of 4.0 and 3.7. Although he was not yet sure what he would do professionally, he told me that being successful for him meant becoming the CEO or founder of a large company.

His ambition was alloyed with hesitation and self-doubt. He doubted his ability to succeed in the terms he had chosen. Often, he expressed that he felt like he did not belong at such an elite institution because his peers were simply better than him. He lamented the loss of his status from being in the top 1% in his high school to being merely average in college. When he felt frustrated by his own perceived mediocre performance, he often became critical of his own goals, stating that happiness was more important than material success and good grades.

He frequently compared himself with his peers and found himself lacking. He felt that his peers were smarter, more disciplined, and more socially savvy than he was. His habit of social comparison was complicated by the fact that his Asian, working-class background often landed him in the minority of any group at this predominantly white and wealthy institution. He felt not only isolated but also disadvantaged compared with his peers. He perceived that his peers mostly came from elite preparatory schools and often had parents who could use their social connections to provide them with the perfect internship. John, in comparison, came from a working-class Chinese background; his parents were first-generation immigrants who had come to the United States and started a laundry business. He felt that he did not have the same advantages as his peers, despite the fact that they were all being judged by the same standard. His habit of social comparison and his relatively disadvantaged background often left him feeling not only isolated but also somewhat resentful about the social injustice.

His interaction with peers was characterized by a deep yearning to win the approval of others coupled with a sensitivity to slights and perceived acts of rejection. He recalled an incident in which a group of friends had made ramen noodles as a late-night snack and invited John to join in. In the hullabaloo of the group, his friends had forgotten to get John a bowl and a spoon for the ramen. John felt excluded, slighted, and consequently resentful of his friends' lack of consideration. He described his friends as being amused by his perceived social awkwardness or "weirdness." He felt that they laughed at him.

His work ethic and creativity were his most valued strengths. In high school, John had joined a summer program for students interested in business, entailing a final team competition requiring development of a business proposal. The proposals were judged based on the quality of the idea and the quality of the presentation. John had the signature vision for both the business and the presentation, and his team eventually won the competition. He described his experience of teamwork and creative triumph as one of the best moments of his life—he felt both genuinely understood and valued by his peers.

John is the son of Chinese immigrants who owned a nail salon in rural Pennsylvania. He has one younger sister with whom he has a good relationship. He described both his parents as hardworking and caring but also quite volatile—prone to angry, uncontrolled outbursts of rage. His father emigrated from mainland China to the United States and started a laundry business. John described him as a quiet and even submissive man, especially toward Americans.

Although the household was mostly calm and supportive, John's father lost control and was violent at times because of marital or familial conflict. When John was barely in elementary school, his father grew angry at John's mother and picked up a plate from the dining room table and smashed it on the wall. Similarly, John described his mom as caring but also volatile. When John was a teenager, he and his mother had a verbal spat that ended with her breaking a picture frame over a chair in an expression of rage. There were instances of violence between the parents; once while in elementary school, John called the police in order to maintain a sense of safety. He described feeling terrified as a child, witnessing his parents' uncontrolled displays of emotion coupled with destructive behavior.

Another salient feature of John's relationship to his parents was their focus on his academic achievement. He recalled an incident when he was in elementary school and received a 93% on an exam. After revealing this to his parents, he was faced with angry criticism for not doing better on the exam. He stated that his parents criticized him for not doing his chores or for disappointing their expectations. Their reproaches often took the form of verbal attacks in which they referred to John as "stupid" of "worthless" or in a variety of other degrading terms. He felt both pained and infuriated by his parents' insults, wanting to win their approval but also to express his superiority to them.

John shared with me that throughout middle school he had been bullied and often made fun of for being overweight and having acne. In high school, he often felt very socially outcast and awkward. He learned to compensate for the humiliations and pains of the social sphere by emphasizing his triumphs in the academic sphere. He thought that though he was socially inferior, he was superior in terms of academic performance.

John suffered from social anxiety as well as issues related to self-esteem. His symptoms had worsened since he gained independence in college, took on a very heavy course load, and began dealing with the stress of transitioning to a different peer group. He felt uncomfortable expressing his feelings toward people and at times felt resentful of people's insensitivity toward him. Despite his high achievements, considerable talents, and generally likable nature, he felt flawed and constantly doubted his self-worth. He was introspective and self-reflective, and showed a self-effacing sense of humor that made him quite likable.

John received psychiatric care while in high school from a private psychiatrist, who had given what John called "talk therapy," but he was not sure about the particular modality or any specific gains he had made as a result. He had no history of inpatient psychiatric treatment and denied any history of suicide attempts or self-injurious behavior. He was born full-term without complications and he met his developmental milestones on time. Throughout school he often excelled in classes and had a select group of close friends. He had no medical problems or allergies. He denied any formal family history of psychiatric illness but stated that it was possible his grandmother suffered from undiagnosed depression. He endorsed a network of social supports, including his family and a few peers. He had had no romantic or intimate relationships, although he did admit to having had crushes on girls in high school. He enjoyed video games and superhero movies. Although he was not raised in any particular religious tradition, he often found guidance in lessons and teaching from the Buddhist tradition.

FORMULATION

From a psychodynamic perspective, John has two core issues: one related to overwhelming experiences of parental anger that underpins his social anxiety and one about regulating his self-esteem that further contributes to his difficulty with social interactions. I used Gabbard's (2014) theoretical framework of social anxiety as resulting from overwhelming childhood experiences of parental rage leading to avoidance of personal anger to explore John's early painful experiences as well as his own aggressive fantasies toward others. I framed John's difficulty regulating his self-esteem using Summers and Barber's (2012) conceptualization of the core psychodynamic problem of low self-esteem.

John had a difficult time being conscious of his own emotions, undermining his ability to become close with others. He projected his anger onto those around him, often guessing, without much corroborating evidence, that others were critical, judgmental, and generally disapproving of him. He was racked with anxiety about other people thinking he was awkward, dumb, or odd. His early frightening experiences of his parents' anger made it difficult for him to own his anger, so he lent it to others to give it back to him in a steady stream of judgments, slights, and criticisms.

Social anxiety, however, was not John's only issue. It became clear within months that he had a difficult time regulating his self-esteem; he felt either superior to others or, more frequently, inferior to them. A common theme in our conversations was John's propensity to compare himself with others. He constantly compared his status with that of his peers—whether he was as smart, disciplined, or talented as they were. He came into the office with worries regarding his grades, class rankings, and ability to be accepted into various elite clubs. Although the competitive and meritocratic culture of John's university might account for some of this, John seemed to have a particular vulnerability to personalizing the institution's mores.

As our conversations continued, another side of John emerged. He felt secretly superior to his peers. His sense of superiority expressed itself in both direct and indirect ways. Directly, John enjoyed talking about his ambitions and confidence and said that his average performance stemmed from his being the son of working-class Chinese immigrants and his lack of opportunity that others had. Beneath what seemed like a pervasive sense of inferiority, John actually thought he was more talented and harder working than his peers but was held back by economic and racial prejudice.

John had considerable strengths of character that were inseparable from his difficulties. I used the technique of strength spotting as described by P. Alex Linley and George Burns (2009). John's most noticeable character strengths included curiosity, persistence, appreciation of beauty, and playfulness. His love of learning shone through in our sessions; he told me about explorations into books, Wikipedia articles, or YouTube channels. Yet, his curiosity was overshadowed by his need to achieve in order to compensate for his damaged sense of self.

John was clearly industrious and persistent, often increasing his effort in the face of academic difficulty. He took on too many courses and activities, spent nearly every hour of his week working, and at times even disregarded his basic needs to eat or sleep. John loved art and design. He enjoyed drawing and creating compositions, but he did not prioritize these activities. Instead, he took courses to support a more prestigious major that was less enjoyable to him. He was very humorous and playful, often making a self-deprecating joke or creatively displaying the magnetic desk toys in the office. Despite his obvious love of play, however, John's extracurricular activities consisted of work for pay and social clubs for networking purposes. He seemed to like play but not value it.

John's strengths were distorted by his core psychodynamic problem of self-esteem. His love of learning, persistence, appreciation of beauty, and playfulness were overshadowed by an intense need to achieve and compensate for an internal sense of self-damage or injury. Avoiding his signature strengths led to a lack of positive emotions in his life, because he did not genuinely enjoy many of his activities. Furthermore, it was hard for him to become engaged in his work because he was often working for the extrinsic reward of a grade instead of working for the intrinsic reward of learning. Lastly, since John had both a dearth of positive emotions and a lack of engagement, he questioned the significance of academic achievement and doubted the ultimate meaning behind the life he had chosen.

COURSE OF TREATMENT

The treatment had two distinct stages: one addressing his social anxiety and the other directed at his dichotomous sense of self. Initially, I noticed that when John told me about painful memories, his tone was cold and intellectual, and his affect was remote, as if he were merely explaining a formula. At times, he even chuckled while talking about being yelled at and belittled by his parents. I pointed out the subtle incongruence in his sad stories and his stoic countenance.

John's stories often evoked feelings of anger or sadness within me; however, I noticed that as he spoke he did not seem particularly angry or sad. I gently pointed this incongruence out to him. We often spoke about how he experienced his own emotions as unpredictable and explosive in the same fashion he experienced his parents' emotions. As the therapeutic alliance built, John slowly began to feel more comfortable expressing his emotions during therapy. At times, he had tears in his eyes when he talked about being subject to his parents' unrelenting standards, unpredictable anger, and emotional distance. At other times, he recalled arguments with his parents with a palpable sense of anger and hostility toward them.

To explore his relationship to anger, we spent quite a bit of time exploring his early experiences of parental anger. We focused on how his parents' explosive and even violent outbursts of anger likely frightened John, making him wary of aggression in others and, crucially, in himself. He experienced anger and, by extension, any feelings as potentially threatening and dangerous. As a result, he learned to cut himself off from his inner feeling states and to focus instead on his intellect and thought processes. John had a difficult time owning his anger and using it in a productive manner. He would ignore slights against him until he became overwhelmed and hurt by even small discourtesies.

By experiencing powerful feelings in the holding environment of therapy, John was able to develop the strength of emotional intelligence and understand that feelings were not the same as actions. He began to learn that anger and hostility can be felt and experienced without consequent hurtful or violent behavior. Although he still struggled with some measure of self-consciousness, he began to feel more comfortable expressing himself in his classes and showed objective improvements on social anxiety scales.

The second focus of the treatment course was on John's self-esteem dysregulation, which often left him feeling overtly inferior to others, with a hidden sense of superiority. The initial phase of therapy entailed eliciting and making explicit John's sense of inferiority—reflecting back to him how he often spoke about himself in denigrating and demeaning terms. We explored this sense of inferiority and his propensity to denigrate himself and connected these experiences to being yelled at and called names by his parents. He internalized these experiences, thinking of himself as someone worthy of insults. John repeated these experiences in the present; when he did not perform up to his own standards, he insulted and criticized himself.

After John became more aware of self-criticism, we began working on exploring his need for superiority and self-idealization. For example, when he had difficulty, he often devalued academic performance, which he otherwise idealized. He told me "none of this stuff matters anyway." His experience of struggling with a large course load was translated to criticism of the culture of success and the competitive meritocracy of his school. At other times of stress, he would immerse himself in Buddhist spirituality and mental training. During these sessions our conversation would focus on his sense of equanimity and acceptance toward all outcomes in his life. Academic performance and material success were nothing compared to spiritual enlightenment and personal happiness. His discounting of the values of the university community served as a means to preserve and even boost his self-esteem: he might not be the best student, but due to his spiritual beliefs he was enlightened and thus superior to those around him.

I began to point out to John that he seemed to have two sides to his personality: one side that felt lesser than everyone and another that felt better than everyone. During one session, we talked about how he often felt empty and hollow on the inside. I expressed my empathy with how painful it must be for him to experience himself in such radically different and opposing ways. He resonated with the notion of being split in two and feeling fragmented. I offered him some hope by stating that although he experienced himself as fragmented and empty, I could see that he was whole and merely struggling with strong feelings.

I pointed out that although he was not perfect socially or academically, he was genuinely intelligent, humorous, and kindhearted. I told him that I was impressed by his diligence and work ethic in taking on a challenging course load, while both working and belonging to several clubs. I celebrated his sense of humor by laughing at his jokes and engaging in banter with him. When he told me about his interest in design and computer programming, I reflected back his natural curiosity and love of learning. He often played with a group of magnetic cubes that could be configured into various shapes that I had on a table near his chair. Although I worried that this would distract from our session, I chose to let him play in order to demonstrate my appreciation for his playfulness.

Despite pointing out his strengths and showing that I valued him as a person, I was careful not to mirror John's perfectionistic standards of himself. In response to his self-criticism, I pointed out that his flaws made him a human being who deserved to be valued and loved. John slowly grasped the notion that he was neither all bad nor all good but an amalgam of both. During one of those sessions while we were talking about his split sense of self, John grew tearful and silent. When I asked him how he felt, he continued to stare at the ground and slowly told me softly that he felt like he could learn to love himself.

John recalled an instance when his mother berated him. He recalled the anger and even open hostility he felt toward her while also recounting how difficult it was to express his anger when he was a young child who was so dependent on his mother. During those moments, when he felt so small and humiliated but also enraged, he learned to regulate both his anger and his self-esteem by directing his anger toward striving to be better than his parents. Although they could insult and belittle him, he would be smarter, more accomplished, and more successful than they were. He told me that he felt guilty about his hostility toward the people who loved him. I empathized with how overwhelmed, vulnerable, and confused John felt as a child when the people who loved and cared for him also belittled and denigrated him.

I framed his split idealized and devalued self, coupled with his fantasy of being better than his parents, as a way of coping with his sense of vulnerability and the complex emotions he felt but likely could not articulate as a child. The outcome for these sessions was surprising. Although John would at times express a sense of inner emptiness, after these sessions he would feel deeply vulnerable and filled with emotion, often tearing up and even crying before leaving. He expressed his bemusement at this newfound state, often asking me, "Why do I feel this way?" or "Why do I feel so sad?"

I was careful neither to overly reassure him and thus take away his sense of vulnerability nor to leave him struggling with this new emotional state by himself. I would answer his questions by offering the suggestion that perhaps for the first time in his life he was sympathizing with himself instead of devaluing or idealizing himself. We further discussed the possibility that his sense of inner emptiness was starting to be filled with an emotional core that he had previously largely ignored. Because he had not dealt with these emotions since he was a child, experiencing them made him feel just as vulnerable as a kid.

Because John's core problem was self-esteem regulation, I chose to repeatedly point out John's genuine character strengths and question his self-criticism and self-idealization. By drawing attention to John's strengths, I aimed to reframe John's self-image from a split superior or inferior sense of self to a more whole and well-integrated one. By becoming more cognizant of his own strengths and the ways in which he could be valued as a whole person with both his strengths and his flaws, he was able to develop a healthier self-image and better manage his self-esteem.

I considered assigning John a gratitude exercise as a means of shifting his attention from his sense of inferiority toward others and as a reliable way to generate positive emotions. Ultimately, I decided not to focus on this technique initially because although it would likely boost John's overall positive emotions and his ability to appreciate the good aspects of his life, it would not directly help in addressing his core problem of low self-esteem. The advantage of focusing on his character strengths was twofold: first, it allowed John to develop a healthier sense of himself, and second, it allowed him to experience more positive emotions and develop more positive relationships.

Outcome

As treatment continued, John became more open to his own vulnerability and his occasional shortcomings. Although he continued to be very demanding of himself, he became more accepting of the occasional subpar grade or class performance. He developed a sense of perspective on his achievements, stating that although it was important to get good grades, this was not the thing that defined him. This perspective allowed him to experience his course work from a place of intrinsic curiosity instead of an extrinsic need to achieve. He pursued changing his major from computer programming to digital design in order to explore his creative and imaginative side.

By making John's defense of idealization/devaluation more conscious and flexible, I also encouraged him to access his own sense of humanity. By questioning his perfectionistic assumptions and having him think through applying his own standards to others, he began to dampen both his self-criticism and his self-idealization. This process helped John bolster his capacity for compassion, forgiveness, and love. Initially, he would tear up about his early childhood experiences as he felt a sense of compassion for his childhood self. As we unpacked the story of his parents' unrelenting standards and his own sense of vulnerability, he began to forgive himself for his own perceived flaws. As his propensity for idealization/devaluation weakened, he began to feel more at ease relating to himself and others as human beings who were both valuable and flawed. This ability to appreciate his own character and that of others from a holistic rather than split stance increased his capacity to love and be loved.

TAKE-HOME POINTS

- Positive psychology interventions can be blended seamlessly with psychodynamic psychotherapy.

- Positive psychology interventions can be tailored to fit the personality structure of each individual patient.

- Patients with difficulty regulating self-esteem may require mirroring of their authentic self and the avoidance of idealization in order to effectively identify and work with their strengths.

REFERENCES

Gabbard GO: Psychodynamic Psychiatry in Clinical Practice. Washington, DC, American Psychiatric Publishing, 2014

Linley PA, Burns GW: Strengthspotting: finding and developing client resources in the management of intense anger, in Happiness, Healing, Enhancement: Your Casebook Collection for Applying Positive Psychology in Therapy. Edited by Burns GW. New York, Wiley, 2009, pp 3–14

Summers RF, Barber JP: Psychodynamic Therapy: A Guide to Evidence-Based Practice. New York, Guilford, 2012

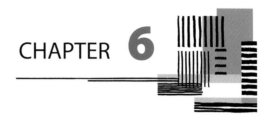

CHAPTER 6

Positivity in the Treatment of Opioid Addiction and Trauma

Margot Montgomery O'Donnell, M.D.

Editors' Introduction

This moving case history of a young woman with medical problems, pain, and opiate addiction demonstrates the application
of positive psychiatry principles to the treatment of trauma and
addiction. The author spells out in detail the positive interventions employed and articulates very clearly the relationship between these interventions and the traditional interventions, both
psychosocial and medical, for these problems. A discussion of
positivity as an antidote to physician burnout adds to the richness
of the clinical picture.

SUMMARY

Meredith is a 26-year-old woman with anxiety, depression, and opiate dependence. Her treatment had two distinct phases. In the first, the goal was symptom
suppression and substance abstinence. The therapeutic interventions reflected
a medical, psychoeducational, and supportive stance. The therapy was adequate
in delivery and response but, in retrospect, unanimated and at times opposi-
tional. Things changed when Meredith accepted inpatient treatment for her
substance dependence. Since Meredith became sober, her second phase of treat-

ment has involved working together in a positive psychiatry model to build skills and a new sense of self and to set goals built on, but not limited to, sobriety.

Person

Chief Complaint and Presentation

Meredith was referred by her primary care doctor following a crisis in the doctor-patient relationship. In her early teens, she suffered a series of hospitalizations and surgeries. Each consecutive intervention was accompanied by high-dose opiate pain management in the hospital and lower-dose prescribing after discharge. Before she met me, Meredith's symptoms had been stable for a few years, but her pain, and her opiate prescriptions, remained. Her physician, a colleague with a reputation for treating complicated young adults, worked with her for almost a decade, but after her third request for additional pills in as many months, the doctor refused to continue prescribing the strong pain medications without psychiatric involvement.

Meredith presents as mature for her age. She describes her medical history, as well as her emotional life, in a clear but clinical style. She states she is a "happy person" who perseveres despite all the obstacles she faces. Meredith has never previously seen a psychiatrist or therapist. She and her family view her struggles as entirely resulting from her medical illness. She attends a local university through the part-time studies department because her illness prevented a traditional college experience. She works afternoons and weekends in a nursing home because it gives her time to study. She resolutely denies being "an addict."

History

Meredith is the only daughter and youngest child in a military family. She moved six times before she was 13 years old. Her mother was a teacher and homemaker and her father a decorated army officer prior to retirement. Meredith was 15 years old when she was first hospitalized for stomach pain and weight loss. Her description of her illness is marked by the injustice of putting her life on hold for treatment, and by several incidents when the medical team failed to care for her. Specifically, she recounts when her nurse shared details of her surgery with her boyfriend's mother. Within days, the information was "all over the school" and the boyfriend broke up with her. Meredith reports having felt a similar sense of violation each time doctors or medical residents in the emergency room failed to acknowledge her pain or offer her "the right" medications. There is a family history of alcoholism on Meredith's maternal side.

After the initial evaluation, I collaborated with Meredith's family and her primary care doctor. I drafted a plan she could use with her physician to decrease her daily opiate dosage by 10% every 2–3 days. The plan would take almost 6 weeks, during which time Meredith needed to take final exams. Alternatively, I offered to take over her prescribing. Meredith decided to work with me. We made a plan to use both psychotherapy and medication to manage her anxiety, depression, and withdrawal. I converted her full pain regimen to the single medication Suboxone, which contains a combination of buprenorphine and naloxone. Buprenorphine is an opiate that, when used as prescribed, offers relief from opiate withdrawal symptoms without a significant cognitive or emotional "high." I prescribed an antidepressant and then a low-dose atypical antipsychotic to manage her anxiety and sadness.

We started exploratory psychotherapy that mostly included weekly management of stresses in school and at work. Meredith completed her semester and tolerated several decreases in her Suboxone. On one occasion, her mother called with concerns that opiates were missing from the house. Meredith denied taking them. On another occasion, she could not tolerate the withdrawal symptoms following a decrease in dosage. We agreed to increasing back to the previous dosage; however, because of legal restrictions on opiate medications, neither the pharmacy nor her insurance company would authorize additional pills. Meredith was angry. She was angry at the doctors who first started her opiates, angry at her primary disease, and now angry at me for taking the medication away. She addressed me in a quiet, seething tone, insisting that my job was to help her, not make her feel worse.

It took several weeks in therapy to repair the sense of betrayal. Meredith and I discussed her hypersensitivity to physical pain and her fear that pain is unending and intolerable, and she persisted with her detoxification. She completed her exams successfully and became opiate free. Over that summer, she was unexpectedly offered a full-time job working for a health care management group. She took the position and, by the fall, was managing several accounts while also taking senior-level courses required for her major.

Unfortunately, Meredith suffered what many recovering opiate addicts call post-acute withdrawal. Traditional opiate withdrawal occurs 2–3 days after last use and includes painful body aches, nausea, diarrhea, sweating, and hopelessness. In contrast, *post-acute withdrawal*, which is not a medical diagnosis, refers to symptoms of malaise, depression, irritability, low motivation, and cognitive "fogginess," which occur or recur for several weeks or months. Meredith was committed to performing well at work. Her new schedule left little time for psychotherapy, which, in retrospect, might have helped us identify and intervene on the risks for relapse. After 2 months of her struggling, Meredith and I decided to restart the Suboxone.

I was away on vacation when I received several calls from Meredith, her mother, and her primary care doctor. Meredith had been using higher Suboxone doses than prescribed and, as she knew from the previous experience, could not get an early refill. In desperation, she altered an old prescription. The pharmacy was suspicious and, after confirming the forgery with her physician, notified the police. Everyone involved agreed the best course of action was immediate inpatient drug and alcohol treatment, and Meredith was admitted that evening.

She took a medical leave from school and left her job. After 30 days of detoxification and rehabilitation, Meredith was again opiate free, but her confidence was shaken. She was becoming aware of all the ways she had used opiate medications over the years: to numb pain but also her emotions, to take on more work than she could manage, to detach from disappointments, and to mask her vulnerabilities. She could not return to her primary care doctor. I agreed to continue working with her on the condition that our goals and our relationship fundamentally change.

FORMULATION

Summers and Barber (2012) identify six common core psychodynamic problems. Meredith presents with the core problem of trauma. She did not suffer an assault, engage in combat, or live through a natural disaster. Instead, she was traumatized by her illness and the myriad of necessary but painful interventions required to treat her. The violation was magnified each time caregivers, who were supposed to protect her, broke her trust or failed to relieve her pain.

Trauma is any event in which a person feels helpless in the face of a threat to self or others. The most severe reactions are diagnosed as posttraumatic stress disorder. Survivors suffer from a collection of symptoms; they experience increased emotional and physical sensitivity to risk (hypervigilance), avoidance of danger and reminders of trauma, and mood swings, including anger, anxiety, and hopelessness. These changes make sense evolutionarily, as they may make an individual more prepared for future threats. However, they greatly impair and impede daily life when the danger has passed and is unlikely to occur again.

Problems

Meredith is hypersensitive to physical pain. She experiences it as a reminder of her past and a threat to her future. Prior to recovery, she used opiates to eliminate even normal, everyday aches and avoid the accompanying fear. She struggles with trust and is constantly vigilant for signs that someone will betray her. In drug and alcohol treatment, secret keeping is considered central to addiction. Participants in Alcoholics Anonymous (AA) often say, "You are as sick as your secrets." This is not only because people in addiction lie about their drug use. For Meredith, being honest makes her feel vulnerable in a world full of people who will hurt or fail to help her. She is angry and sad about all the ways her illness made her life harder. She sees missing school, losing her boyfriend, even developing her addiction as all caused by her illness. Her losses are all the more poignant because like many trauma survivors, she has a sense of a foreshortened future. She does not imagine her life progressing the same way for her as it will for her peers. Sometimes, she cannot envision a future at all.

Strengths

Meredith identifies closely with her father and the quiet strength of his military service. She is intelligent, an accomplished student, and an exceptionally hard worker. She practiced resilience and flexibility with each childhood relocation and hospitalization. She makes friends easily, whether at a new school, job, or medical facility. Like many people who have faced trauma, she is sensitive to the suffering of others.

INTERVENTIONS

Meredith's psychotherapy shifted dramatically after she left rehabilitation. Her treatment regimen now includes weekly sessions with an addiction counselor, a women's therapy group, and a family therapist. Therapy goals are well defined and shared freely between collaborating providers and Meredith's family. Our weekly sessions follow a pattern of reviewing the previous week's events, identifying and processing difficult emotions or interactions, and then setting goals for the upcoming week.

Gratitude

Gratitude is one of the best-researched positive interventions. Regularly directing attention to the good things in life has been shown to improve sleep, mood, and overall quality of life (Emmons and McCullough 2004). In her resilience trainings, Dr. Karen Reivich calls practicing gratitude "hunting the good stuff" (Reivich and Shatté 2002). Since leaving rehabilitation, Meredith has struggled with sadness and depression related to the loss of her identity as a student and "good" daughter. The trauma of her medical illness contributes to Meredith's constant focus on risk. We use several practices of gratitude to soften her internal critic and challenge her hypervigilance.

Within a few weeks of discharge from rehabilitation, Meredith felt stuck. She had trouble getting out of bed. She was exhausted after a small number of previously "easy" tasks. She grew disappointed in herself and in sobriety. I challenged Meredith to "hunt the good stuff" by keeping a daily list of successes. Some days staying clean is all she can accomplish. Other days she lists showering, calling friends, attending treatment, or spending time with family. For a previously hard-driving, results-oriented woman, this adjustment is disorienting. Her stoic, military-minded family similarly struggles to identify and be grateful for reasonable accomplishments. Practicing gratitude for sobriety helps Meredith, and her family, minimize disappointment by focusing on the present and the progress she has made.

Meredith also struggles to tolerate physical discomfort in recovery. Aches and pains feel abnormal after years of opiate exposure. Many sensations trigger memories of her illness and lead to fear of recurring disease. In session, we label this *hypervigilance*. As a combat veteran might scan rooftops for snipers, Meredith surveys her body for potential threats. We discuss how emotionally and mentally exhausting it is to stay on guard all the time. This metaphor in particular helps Meredith feel less ashamed. With less shame and embarrassment, she is able to push herself to exercise and socialize more. We then use session time to make note of sensations that do not progress to recurrence. Finally, we augment this traditional exposure intervention with a gratitude exercise.

Hypervigilance is the act of overfocusing on risk. We attempt to counteract this attention by consciously focusing on security. Each time Meredith has back pain or feels fatigue, she makes a list of what feels good in her body or what she has accomplished physically. Her list includes sleeping through the night (without medication), walking the trail behind her house, and eating a good meal. These are all things she identifies her body doing for her, instead of to her or against her. It is a subtle intervention, but seems to be helping Meredith live more fully in her own skin.

Positive Communication

Trauma leaves many victims having lifetime challenges in establishing and maintaining trust. Gratitude helps Meredith to trust her body after grave illness. However, addiction is a family disease. Meredith's mood swings, secrecy, stealing, and lying nearly crippled her parents' ability to trust her. Meredith's trauma also makes it hard for her to fully trust them. Rebuilding the relationship is a slow and sometimes bumpy process.

Since her surgeries in high school, Meredith has had to rely heavily on her parents for physical and financial support. Although she is grateful, she also craves privacy. Her parents, who were caught off guard by the severity and frequency of her addiction, want transparency and reassurance that she is sober. Meredith needed her mom's daily support during her illness.

During her addiction, while she was lying about the drug use, she relied heavily on her mom's advice and direction in school and work. Meredith now experiences her mom's inquiries as criticism. She withdraws and shares less. Her parents worry that she is using drugs again and become more intrusive. The cycle hurts their ability to enjoy and support each other.

Resilience programs such as the Penn Resiliency Program and Master Resilience Training (Revich and Seligman 2011) and therapies such as dialectical behavior therapy (Linehan 2015) offer scripts for healthy communication. Models like DEAL teach the following: **D**escribing a situation, **E**xpressing emotional concerns, **A**sking for input before **A**sking for change, and **L**isting the responses or consequences. After Meredith is taught the script, she is able to apply it to small, everyday conversations with her parents as well as more meaningful negotiations.

In one session, Meredith presented with anger after a fight with her mother. Her mom wanted to know why she had come in late the night before. She expressed anger at Meredith for keeping her bedroom messy and accused her of not doing enough to get back to school. Meredith felt like no one recognized how hard she was working on her sobriety. After identifying these themes in therapy, we used the DEAL script to plan for the next encounter. A week later, when a similar conflict occurred, Meredith was tempted to shut down and "just 'yes' her to death." Instead, she told her mom that she got in late because she was at a meeting. She shared how her anxiety often prevented her from hanging out after AA meetings, so it felt like a success for her to stay out a little longer. She asked about her mom's biggest concern. Her mom grew tearful explaining that she always worried about relapse when Meredith was out of the house. She stays awake until she believes Meredith is safe for the night. Together, they agreed that Meredith would text anytime she would be out later than 11:00 P.M. and wake her mom once she arrived home. Both mother and daughter were satisfied, if not happy, with the negotiation. I joked with Meredith that this is the true sign of a good compromise.

Values and Strengths

Now 9 months without drugs, Meredith is planning to return to school. However, she has rescheduled several meetings with her dean and missed the deadline to register for classes. I interpret this behavior as avoidance, which is common in the trauma formulation. Meredith then endorses significant anxiety about school. Previously, when she faced a work or academic deadline, she used opiates to manage the stress. Without them, she is afraid of failing. Worse, she is afraid of being a failure. By exploring this idea of identity, Meredith is able to verbalize the double bind she used for years to rationalize her drug use and protect her ego.

Meredith describes how the opiates decreased her anxiety, increased her energy, and helped her push through pain to complete papers and projects. At first, she believed she was just "leveling the playing field." She "deserved" to work pain free like everybody else. She progressed to justifying the pills because she had lost so much time due to her illness. Eventually, she needed the drugs to mask how overwhelmed she had become with school, work, and family commitments. She would then turn around and use her multiple commitments and good grades to "prove" to herself, her family, and her doctors that she could not possibly be an addict. She was "functioning so well!"

From being walked through the insidious trap of identity and addiction, Meredith gained enormous insight. However, she now needs a concrete plan to "avoid avoidance" and get back to school. Peterson and Seligman (2004) describe 24 personal strengths that describe how people behave at their best. On the Values in Action Survey (Peterson and Park 2009), Meredith's signature strengths were identified as judgment, perseverance, and perspective. We are now using these strengths to help her plan new ways of managing anxiety about school. The goal is to form a new identity with health, sobriety, and authenticity at the core.

Peterson and Seligman (2004) defines *judgment* as considering a decision analytically and being willing to change opinions. We lean into Meredith's *judgment* by using lots of cognitive therapy skills such as making pro/con lists and challenging assumptions. When Meredith is reluctant to email the dean about reenrolling, we write out the risks and benefits. The worst that can happen is that she does not reenroll (exactly the situation she is in currently and managing well). Meredith can tolerate the worst-case scenario because of her strong *perspective*. She can see things from several angles and appreciate the big picture. Due to her trauma, not in spite of it, Meredith is in the unique position to know what really qualifies as "life or death."

Finally, and unsurprisingly, Meredith finds power in *perseverance*. Peterson and Park's (2009) two-prong description of perseverance includes effort to complete a task and endurance to continue in spite of challenges. Identifying Meredith's "Superwoman" complex is an important first step. We agree together that moving forward she will need to draw her self-esteem from her effort, not her outcomes. She may be a B student without opiates, but by using perspective she can identify that being a sober B student is more valuable and more sustainable than being an addicted A student. Hard work is a superpower too!

Optimism

Substance dependence is a complex disorder with no single cause or cure. Trauma likely plays a role in increasing vulnerability to substance use. Medical traumas such as Meredith's are especially risky due to accompanying prescription pain management. On the flip side, once people with addiction begin using illicitly, they are more likely to experience trauma. Overdose is an incredibly scary experience, both for the person experiencing it and for the witness. The illegal status of substances invites exposure to crime and the criminal justice system, physical and sexual violence, and financial stresses such as job loss and homelessness. These experiences can lead people with addiction and trauma to share many traits, including a sense of foreshortened future.

Hopelessness is a challenge to all treatment. A patient's expectation that she can change may be the single most important factor in treatment engagement and success. However, if death feels looming, hope can be hard to muster. Seligman (2006) discusses optimism as a cognitive assumption, or an attributional style. People are not optimistic or pessimistic. They have a habit of thinking that focuses on their own contribution to good outcomes (optimism) or bad (pessimism) as well as the role of luck in bad outcomes (optimism) or good (pessimism).

Meredith struggles to make long-term plans. She experiences enormous anxiety about a particular grade or a specific fight with her mother, but she seldom talks about bigger life goals of partnering or profession. Her treatment is unique for a woman in her 20s for its lack of content about marriage or children. When I pointed this out to Meredith, she identified having trouble imagining and taking actions toward her future even prior to her opiate use. After her second surgery, she had a bad reaction to anesthesia and almost died. Since then, she has had trouble imagining life past 30. I introduced attributional styles to combat Meredith's underlying belief that her future is out of her control. In AA meetings, participants frequently recite the serenity prayer, which asks God for the serenity to accept things that are unchangeable and strength to make change where possible. Both ideas serve to increase optimism about the future by focusing on personal responsibility.

When Meredith grows overwhelmed by the steps ahead of her, we use a weekly calendar to identify concrete actions she can take. We work together to ensure that each week includes activities focused on the aspects of her life she most wants to improve—sobriety, relationships, and school. She is exerting agency in the areas of her life she wants to grow in. That leaves less energy for her to worry about fate, while building a foundation that can support a real future.

Positive Interventions for the Psychiatrist

I once had a supervisor describe practicing psychotherapy as "intoxicating." Like a drug, a good session makes me feel connected, insightful, and valuable. But also like a drug, there are real risks to overuse. Mental health care providers suffer a high rate of burnout and compassion fatigue. Drug and alcohol treatment providers in particular work unpredictable hours with a sick population and may suffer trauma of their own when patients relapse, disappear, or die.

Positive psychology is rooted in the premise that human accomplishments, values, behaviors, and relationships are important for happiness. When therapeutic success is measured by what a patient can refrain from doing, like using drugs or feeling sad, the therapist risks exhaustion trying to prevent bad behavior. Positive psychology, alternatively, lets the therapist act like a coach. The role is to offer ideas and provide a safe environment in which to practice and fail. Negative feelings and behaviors are understood as part of the course of treatment, as learning opportunities. And the patient's success or failure belongs to the patient alone.

The nation is in the grips of an opiate epidemic. In 2015, more than 33,000 Americans died of opiate overdose (Rudd et al. 2016). Many patients, like Meredith, are first exposed in medical settings. Health care providers have a duty to provide quality addiction care to meet the growing need. Positive psychiatric practices offer patients concrete skills and foster hope for recovery. Positive psychiatric practices also help therapists to combat compassion fatigue by increasing their own self-care.

I try to record my daily gratitudes, and I succeed some of the time. I practice acceptance of my failings, including forgetting to record my gratitudes. I work on honesty in my relationships as well as asking for help, though here I fall short too. I review my signature strengths when making hard decisions and before committing my limited resources to a new activity. I focus on the parts of my life that I can control and improve, which seldom include the behaviors or feelings of my patients. This is freeing. And it keeps me coming back to work.

OUTCOME

Meredith continues to work hard in therapy. Like many people in recovery, she experienced an initial joy and relief, often called "the pink cloud." Now she is facing the hard work of lasting sobriety. She is rebuilding her life for the second time in as many decades. She is sad about her losses and compares herself negatively to her peers. She worries about relapse, both of her medical illness and of her drug use. But she is proud of her progress. She is grateful for her parents' support. She is afraid of not being able to perform academically, but she is excited that she can really own her accomplishments without the disclaimer "I was high."

Meredith struggles to go to recovery meetings. When she attends, however, she often notices the same themes we explore in therapy. Gratitude is front and center, as is acceptance. There is a lot of talk about honesty, with oneself and with others. Relationships are valued. Participants are encouraged to improve old relationships by making amends and build new relationships by helping others in recovery. What AA calls "self-inventory," psychotherapy calls "insight." Maybe most importantly, the 12 Steps codify beliefs and behaviors that make for a good life. Taking away symptoms like sadness, lying, or pain is not the goal. Positive psychology started with the revolutionary idea that mental health could also be about increasing the good instead of, or in addition to, minimizing the bad. Meredith is building a meaningful life and identity with room for illness and imperfection. Therapy, like recovery, is one day at a time.

TAKE-HOME POINTS

- Positive psychiatry is a set of skills that can be offered to patients, as well as a process of delivering therapy.

- Positive interventions such as gratitude, positive communication, signature strengths, and optimism can target specific psychiatric complaints, including symptoms of trauma.

- Taking a positive stance can help therapists focus on the good in their patients and in their own lives, combating compassion fatigue and burnout.

- Positive psychiatry shares similarities with the 12-Step model and therefore is helpful in psychotherapy with patients who have substance dependence.

REFERENCES

Emmons RA, McCullough ME (eds): The Psychology of Gratitude. New York, Oxford University Press, 2004

Linehan MM: DBT Skills Training Handouts and Worksheets. New York, Guilford, 2015

Peterson C, Park N: Classifying and measuring strengths of character, in Oxford Handbook of Positive Psychology, 2nd Edition. Edited by Lopez SJ, Snyder CR. New York, Oxford University Press, 2009, pp 25–33

Peterson C, Seligman ME: Character Strengths and Virtues: A Handbook and Classification, Vol 1. New York, Oxford University Press, 2004

Revich KJ, Seligman ME: Master Resilience Training in the U.S. Army. Am Psychol 66(1)25–34, 2011

Reivich KJ, Shatté A: The Resilience Factor: 7 Essential Skills for Overcoming Life's Inevitable Obstacles. New York, Broadway Books, 2002

Rudd RA, Seth P, David F, et al: Increases in drug and opioid-involved overdose deaths—United States, 2010–2015. MMWR Morb Mortal Wkly Rep 65:1445–1452, 2016 28033313

Seligman ME: Learned Optimism: How to Change Your Mind and Your Life. New York, Vintage Books, 2006

Summers RF, Barber JP: Psychodynamic Therapy: A Guide to Evidence-Based Practice. New York, Guilford, 2012

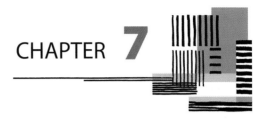

CHAPTER 7

Effective Use of Positive Psychiatry Concepts in the Psychotherapy of an Older Patient Living With Bipolar Disorder

Daniel D. Sewell, M.D.

Yash B. Joshi, M.D., Ph.D.

Editors' Introduction

A long-term treatment that emphasizes positive interventions—acts of kindness, engagement in meaningful activities, employing personal strengths, and counting blessings—allows a middle-aged man to experience a fuller and richer life and helps in buffering losses and the inevitable challenges of aging. This case history shows the importance of strength building for increasing resilience, not only for reducing symptoms.

Summary

When V first sought treatment from one of us (DDS) 20 years ago, he was a 52-year-old single gay man with bipolar II disorder and attention-deficit/hyperactivity disorder (ADHD) with low self-esteem and a number of personality characteristics that provided the foundation for the successful application of positive psychological interventions (PPIs). PPIs are activities designed to promote positive outcomes by employing positive processes (Parks and Biswas-Diener 2013). Research has found that PPIs have the potential to improve the lives of individuals experiencing a spectrum of medical and psychiatric disorders and problems: depression (Seligman et al. 2006; Sin and Lyubomirsky 2009), suicidality (Huffman et al. 2014), schizophrenia (Meyer et al. 2012), nicotine dependence (Kahler et al. 2014), and chronic pain (Hausmann et al. 2014). This case demonstrates the value of PPIs in treating patients with bipolar disorders as well as older adults—two subgroups of patients for which there is currently a relative paucity of information in the scientific literature about the value of PPIs. The patient's psychiatrist, who is board-certified in both adult and geriatric psychiatry, began introducing PPIs while working to establish an optimal psychotropic medication regimen and has continued to employ PPIs since that time. The absence of recurrent mood episodes, the patient's ongoing self-reports of a meaningful and enjoyable life, and his ability to grieve the recent death of his life partner without complications are some of the outcomes that suggest that the use of both psychiatric medications and PPIs is responsible for the patient's improved mental health, mood stability, and overall satisfaction with his life.

PERSON

Presentation and Chief Complaint

At the time of his first appointment 20 years ago, V was a 52-year-old single gay white male social worker, health system administrator for the county in which he was living, and artist. His chief complaint was "I need a new psychiatrist." He explained that he had been receiving mental health care for several decades but because of a change in his insurance, he needed to find a new psychiatrist. He arrived on time for his appointment, which began 20 minutes late. When greeted in the reception area of the clinic, he suggested that his appointment be rescheduled, but the psychiatrist insisted that he remain for his appointment and assured him that the length of his visit would not be abbreviated due to a late start. Throughout the ensuing years, V periodically spoke about how powerfully helpful that moment was for him.

History of the Present Illness

When he was in his early 30s, V divorced his wife and began the process of coming out as a gay man. The psychological challenges associated with this process inspired him, for the first time in his life, to seek out mental health care. He began working with a clinical psychologist. Unfortunately, the psychologist employed methods that were both unconventional and unethical and included arranging for V to date other gay male clients in the therapist's caseload and at least one invitation to the therapist's home, where the therapist encouraged V and a number of the therapist's other gay male clients to sit together naked in a hot tub. V eventually stopped seeing this psychologist, but the psychological injuries experienced while in the care of this therapist have been a focus of his psychotherapy work with DDS. Shortly after ending his relationship with the clinical psychologist, V began working with a psychiatrist who diagnosed him with attention-deficit disorder and major depressive disorder and began prescribing medications and providing supportive psychotherapy and cognitive-behavioral psychotherapy (CBT).

By the time V arrived for his first appointment with DDS, he had been treated with a number of psychotropic medications over his life, but for the past several years he had been doing reasonably well taking a combination of fluoxetine, nortriptyline, methylphenidate, and low-dose alprazolam as needed daily. He was, however, still experiencing disruptive recurrent episodes of depression and hypomania. The initial focus of his work with DDS was managing breakthrough depression symptoms, which responded to incremental increases in his fluoxetine dose. After a period of euthymia, V had an episode of hypomania. This episode led V to recall that he had been experiencing similar episodes since young adulthood but had never recognized them as episodes of abnormal mood. He reported that these episodes lasted weeks to months, usually once or twice a year, and during these episodes he experienced increased goal-directed activity, mood lability, irritability, greater impulsivity, and noticeably increased libido. This newly accessed historical information led to a revision in his mood disorder diagnosis from major depressive disorder to bipolar II disorder. He subsequently had trials of several mood stabilizers, including lithium, which was unsuccessful because of the development of a tremor that was so severe that V could no longer paint. Eight years ago, he began a trial of lamotrigine, which has proven very successful. Since beginning treatment with lamotrigine, he has had rare episodes of mild hypomania, during which he endorsed the above-listed hypomanic symptoms for a few days, as well as several episodes of subsyndromal depressive symptoms lasting a few weeks at a time. He has no history of inpatient psychiatric hospitalizations and has made no suicide attempts, and has now been receiving care from the same psychiatrist for over 20 years. V's substance use history is remarkable only for alcohol use disorder, but he has not met criteria for any substance use disorder for many decades.

V's medical history is notable for hypertension, hypothyroidism, erectile dysfunction, hyperlipidemia, and arthritis. These are currently being treated, respectively, with losartan; levothyroxine; alprostadil-papaverine-phentolamine intracavernosal injection as needed and testosterone gel; simvastatin 40 mg daily; and celecoxib daily. V's family history is notable for alcohol use disorder in his father and his brother. His brother died in middle age from medical complications of alcoholism. In addition, his father had late-onset Alzheimer's disease.

Developmental and Social History

V was the second born of two children and grew up in a household with an emotionally distant father who struggled with alcohol dependence and a mother whom he described as codependent. He was a bright student and did well in school, but his youth was marked by social isolation and bullying because he developed persistent bilateral blepharitis, which caused the rims of his eyes to be swollen and red through his grade school and teenage years and left him feeling defective. He attended college, graduated with a liberal arts degree, and then enlisted in the navy during the Vietnam War. He served three tours on several ships in combat theaters where he would often have to be vigilant and at his station for days at a time, experiencing a near-constant volley of rocket fire. It was during this time that he began to grapple with his sexuality and began to appreciate that he was gay, which left him once again feeling defective, as well as conflicted and ambivalent. He developed a close bond with another enlisted gay man, but their only physical contact was holding hands while on deck during the dead of night for brief moments at a time. He felt a tremendous sense of loss when their tours of duty separated them and he was not able to continue his relationship with this man.

After an honorable discharge from the navy, he obtained a degree in social work and entered the field of public health, eventually becoming a high-level administrator in his county's public health department, advocating for those with developmental disabilities. Although he continued to be conflicted about his sexuality, he met a woman, K, with whom he began a relationship that resulted in an 8-year marriage. V and K were not sexually intimate, but they found platonic intimacy in each other's company, which they both cherished, with V noting that the happiest day of his life was the day he married K.

When he was in his 30s, V came out to K, which ended their marriage, but their separation was amicable. V was pleased that he had finally come out, but he struggled with his identity as a gay man, which led to great difficulty finding meaningful connections, and he fell into cycles of abusive relationships with male partners. Around this time, in the 1980s, many of his friends were falling ill and dying from HIV-associated complications, and V began a period of attending funerals nearly weekly for months on end. He began experiencing persistent depressive symptoms and sought help from several therapists, finding one who specialized in the treatment of gay men. As noted above, this therapist violated the therapeutic frame by arranging for V to participate in a variety of sexual acts with the psychotherapist's other gay patients. Shortly after a series of these experiences, V discontinued his work with this therapist. A while after this, he experienced an episode of depression. He remembered "crying all of the time" and having so many symptoms of depression that he could not work. He then found a psychiatrist who helped him address his depression with medications as well as supportive psychotherapy and CBT. The initial medication that the therapist prescribed was nortriptyline. V stated that after taking this medication for several weeks, he felt on top of the world. In retrospect, it is possible that his robust response to nortriptyline was an antidepressant-associated hypomanic episode.

Eventually, V started an organization where gay professionals could meet, and he started to hold groups and events to support people who were experiencing end-stage HIV-associated illness. He retired in his 50s from the public health department and then began working for a variety of LGBT nonprofits; this work energized him. V joined an Adult Children of Alcoholics (ACA) group, supported men with alcohol use disorder attempting sobriety, and employed them on his property to do odd jobs. V also found peace in aiding both his father and mother as they aged and became infirm, remarking that as his father developed dementia, the two began enjoying each other's company for the first time. V found C, a gay man with whom he felt secure, including during sexual intimacy, and he felt gratified for the first time in a romantic relationship. He also reconnected with K, who, widowed after her second husband died, relied on V to help scrutinize men to date.

As V progressed with therapy through these life changes, he found himself beginning to better appreciate the magnitude of his past losses and traumas, and sought to resolve and move beyond them in therapy. Although he was proud of his past accomplishments, he found himself grappling with issues of stagnation and the cultivation of a personal legacy as he aged. He was happy with C as his partner overall, but C's worsening fibrotic lung disease caused their sexual needs to diverge, which caused some tension in the relationship. He also struggled with reconciling his role as a dutiful son to his parents given the alcoholism and dysfunction that had characterized his family life as far back as he could remember. With these issues in mind, his psychiatrist leveraged the patient's strengths and past history within the frame of positive psychiatry to improve the patient's quality of life, in general, and to reduce his risk of mood episode relapse, in particular.

FORMULATION

Problems

Like those of many patients, especially patients who are older, V's health problems include medical illnesses, psychiatric illnesses, and psychological vulnerabilities. As noted earlier, his psychiatric diagnoses were ultimately determined to be bipolar II disorder and ADHD. Psychologically, he was burdened by low self-esteem, related to his father's lifelong struggle with alcoholism; his chronic blepharitis in childhood; and his membership in an often maligned and misunderstood sexual minority, which had led him into a series of unhealthy relationships in which many of his emotional and sexual needs were not met and in which he overfunctioned.

Strengths

V had a number of strengths, including above-average intelligence, a college education, artistic talents, financial security, and well-honed social skills, including the ability to use kindness strategically to obtain what he needed and wanted from others. He was also psychologically minded, was motivated to achieve a better state of emotional well-being, and had a good sense of humor. As noted above, for a number of years V had been actively involved in ACA and through this experience had learned about healthy communication and healthy relationships.

INTERVENTIONS AND TREATMENT

The initial focus of V's psychiatric care was establishing a psychotropic medication regimen that reduced the frequency and intensity of his mood episodes without causing problematic medication side effects. During this phase of his treatment, he was provided with supportive psychotherapy, and a number of preexisting adaptive personality traits were acknowledged, praised, and encouraged. Deliberately fostering these personality traits and associated behaviors represented the application of the PPI that seeks to increase the patient's engagement in purposeful, meaningful, or enjoyable activities. The success he had helping nonprofit community organizations obtain grant funds, along with external recognition he obtained for these successes, served as reminders for V of his talents and abilities, gave him a sense of purpose, and added meaning to his life. After several failed mood stabilizer trials, the addition of lamotrigine led to a level of mood stabilization that he had never before achieved, and the main focus of his care subsequently shifted from medication trials and medication dose adjustments to psychotherapy with increasing emphasis on PPIs. In addition to the PPI mentioned above, the following PPIs have been a focus of V's psychotherapy: 1) committing acts of kindness, 2) identifying and deliberately employing personal strengths, 3) counting blessings, and 4) savoring.

V's multiple strengths, including his resilience, hardiness, and positive coping style, made him an ideal candidate for the introduction and application of PPIs. These strengths served as fertile ground in which PPIs could take root. PPIs are also helpful for individuals who may not have the number or type of personal strengths of someone like V. For these individuals, the therapist needs to anticipate that adoption and mastery of PPIs may take longer and may require more explanation, in-session rehearsal, and encouragement.

In theory, any of the PPIs employed in the treatment of V could have been introduced at any point during his course of psychotherapy with DDS, but various factors influenced the optimal timing of the introduction and use of certain PPIs. For example, while he was still employed as a health system administrator and simultaneously caring for his aging parents, identifying and employing personal strengths and counting blessings proved to be more congruent with his circumstances and the demands on his time and energy. Reciting his blessings out loud during his psychotherapy sessions and making written lists of his blessings while at home were activities that he was able to integrate into the rhythm of his week and did not require an amount of time or energy that would have been prohibitive given the fullness of his life. As a result, during this phase of his care, these particular PPIs were emphasized. After his retirement and after both of his parents had passed away, we discovered that he had more time and energy for acts of kindness and for savoring. We also discovered that the knowledge, skills, and experiences he had acquired during his career were strengths that he was able to use with great success in helping nonprofit organizations.

Committing Acts of Kindness

V is, by nature, a kind person. During his childhood, he often felt undervalued and unprotected, especially by his parents and his brother. He learned that acts of kindness were one method of building relationships and achieving some degree of physical and emotional safety. Of course, acts of kindness often yield other benefits to the person who is being kind, such as confirming one's sense of mastery, sublimating feelings of helplessness, and inspiring others to be helpful and accommodating in return. As a result, any acts of kindness that V shared during his sessions were celebrated. His acts of kindness sometimes allowed him to employ his personal strengths and actually involved the simultaneous use of two PPIs. For example, his work as a health system administrator helped him become a skillful and successful grant writer. As a result, after he retired from his work as a county administrator, he was able to use his knowledge and experience in this area by assisting a number of local nonprofits in writing and submitting grant proposals.

When V's father developed dementia, as his parents' only surviving child, V became increasingly involved in helping his parents. Once again, his background in social work was a very big asset. He helped his parents access community resources that allowed his father to remain at home much longer than he otherwise could have. Subsequently, when his father could no longer remain at home safely, V helped his mother select a residential community for his father. V was encouraged to discuss these efforts during his appointments and was praised for his knowledge, skills, and generosity.

Identifying and Deliberately Employing Personal Strengths

In addition to PPIs that capitalized on his background and training in social work, PPIs that incorporated his talent as an artist were also employed. V discovered and developed artistic talents in a variety of areas, including watercolor painting, assemblage art, jewelry making, and beading. His skills and talents in these areas provided V with regular opportunities for acknowledgment and validation and served to strengthen his sense of self-worth and self-esteem. In addition, his artistic aptitudes and interests helped strengthen existing relationships. For example, his significant other was also a painter, and he and V enrolled in art classes together. His ability as an artist also helped to expand his social network. For example, V began a friendship with a master beader whom he had met at her art store and studio and then began to meet regularly in either her or his art studio to work on projects in parallel.

Counting Blessings

While in school to become a social worker, and subsequently while a psychotherapy patient, V became acquainted with CBT. His prior knowledge and experience helped him quickly accept the value of regularly reflecting on what was good about his life. During psychotherapy sessions, time was regularly devoted to reminding both of us about the good things in his life, such as his relationship with his life partner, his friends, his financial security, his cozy home located in a safe and pedestrian-friendly neighborhood with a family-owned coffeehouse, his dog, and his team of health care providers. Several times a year, he spontaneously spends time during psychotherapy sessions discussing his gratitude for the care he has received and continues to receive from DDS, in general, and the helpfulness of the initial interaction he had with DDS, in particular. After more than 20 years, he continues to describe how helpful it was that DDS did not reschedule his initial appointment when the appointment got off to a late start. He also talks about how helpful it was that the length of his initial appointment was not shortened due to its tardy start time. These experiences helped him overcome his distrust of mental health care providers while also helping him feel valued and important. Although overtly expressed positive regard and gratitude from a patient may challenge the therapist's own sense of self-worth, each of these moments is met with expressions of happiness that the way his initial encounter with DDS transpired proved to be so helpful.

Savoring

Savoring is a technique that requires a person to observe, acknowledge, describe, and enjoy, as fully as possible, a positive situation or experience in order to benefit contemporaneously from the positive emotions that this moment has authored. The technique of savoring also includes remembering a positive event and/or describing a positive event to another person so that the positive emotions associated with this moment are once again evoked. During V's psychotherapy sessions, there is regular acknowledgment of the importance of being present and of being in the moment. Since his retirement, V has been able to travel to various destinations around the world. While traveling, he strives to be in the moment and to appreciate with all of his senses the new experiences he is having. When he returns, his sessions often become an extension of the savoring process as he shares his memories of his travels and often brings in photos or souvenirs. When he travels, he often spends time painting with watercolors, and he shares these images during his sessions and talks about where he was and what he was doing when he created each painting. These experiences immediately reactivate the positive feelings that he was having while he was traveling and help him avoid feelings of sadness or anxiety.

OUTCOME

The combination of an optimal psychotropic medication regimen and the ongoing and consistent use of PPIs has helped V achieve a level of adaptive functioning and psychological well-being that otherwise might not have been possible. Unfortunately, his life partner recently died from end-stage fibrotic lung disease. V's grief process following this loss has served to spotlight the success of his mental health care and especially the routine manner in which he now employs a variety of PPIs. The loss of his life partner has been challenging but has not triggered a mood episode relapse.

V continues to meet with DDS on a regular basis for combined medication management and psychotherapy appointments and for appointments focused only on psychotherapy. He lives independently in his own home along with two small dogs. He manages a number of investment properties that he inherited from his parents. He does some of the maintenance on these properties himself and hires others to do some of the maintenance work. He has a number of close friends with whom he socializes on a regular basis. For example, he meets one of his friends for a weekly hike, and he has another friend with whom he attends the theater. Over the course of his therapy, he has experienced increased interest in an extended life span. When his therapy began, his day-to-day life was so challenging and uncomfortable that he had no desire for a long life. As his symptoms receded and the quality of his life improved, he began to view his potential longevity in a much more favorable way. He is planning to live at least another 20 years. When he turns 90, he plans to hand over his property management duties to a property management company.

Unlike before he began working with DDS, V now uses PPIs on a regular basis. For example, his recently deceased life partner had a niece who is a member of a sexual minority group, and because of this the niece had a special connection to V and her uncle. V recently made a "memory box" for her to remind her of her uncle and his love for her. He filled the box with a variety of items of her uncle's, including a lock of her uncle's hair. This is one example of an ongoing series of kind acts he shares with others. His work as a property manager allows him to use his personal strengths on a regular basis, such as the assessment skills he acquired during his social work training, which now help him to select desirable tenants. During his psychotherapy sessions, he sets aside time to review with me the things in his life that he counts as blessings, including his supportive and trustworthy friends, his comfortable income, the neighborhood in which he lives, and his psychiatrist. V also regularly savors his life experiences, such as a recent musical play that he attended and then discussed with me during a session. Unlike before his mood was stabilized and he learned about and began using PPIs on a regular basis, he now only very rarely has a day during which psychiatric symptoms impact him in any significant way. He feels rightly proud of the work he has done in psychotherapy and the sustained good health he now enjoys. During a recent psychotherapy session, he reflected on the course of his illness prior to beginning his work with DDS. He stated, "I had to unlearn that a pill was going to fix my life. I had so many [mood episode] relapses." He spoke about how the combination of the right medications, his psychotherapy work with DDS and his use of PPIs, and his ongoing use of concepts acquired through his engagement with ACA, had given him a degree of mood stability and quality of life that he had never before experienced. He has begun learning both French and Spanish and is planning to take piano lessons. As previously noted, he also frequently expresses gratitude to DDS for the care that he has received. In a recent psychotherapy session he explained that at his first appointment with DDS, he perceived that DDS was genuinely interested in him and this "brought me hope."

TAKE-HOME POINTS

- Positive psychological interventions (PPIs) have the potential to improve the health and well-being of individuals struggling with a spectrum of medical and psychiatric illnesses.

- Research has demonstrated that PPIs engender and sustain positive emotions, which in turn help reduce psychiatric symptoms and improve overall quality of life.

- PPIs include acts of kindness; engaging in purposeful, meaningful, or enjoyable activities; identifying and deliberately employing personal strengths; counting blessings; and savoring.

- This case study of an older patient living with bipolar disorder suggests that older adults as well as individuals living with bipolar disorder may benefit from PPIs.

REFERENCES

Hausmann LR, Parks A, Youk AO, et al: Reduction of bodily pain in response to an online positive activities intervention. J Pain 15(5):560–567, 2014 24568751

Huffman JC, DuBois CM, Healy BC, et al: Feasibility and utility of positive psychology exercises for suicidal inpatients. Gen Hosp Psychiatry 36(1):88–94, 2014 24230461

Kahler CW, Spillane NS, Day A, et al: Positive psychotherapy for smoking cessation: treatment development, feasibility and preliminary results. J Posit Psychol 9(1):19–29, 2014 24683417

Meyer PS, Johnson DP, Parks A, et al: Positive living: a pilot study of group positive psychotherapy for people with schizophrenia. J Posit Psychol 7:239–248, 2012

Parks AC, Biswas-Diener R: Positive interventions past, present and future, in Mindfulness, Acceptance and Positive Psychology: The Seven Foundations of Well-Being. Edited by Kashdan T, Ciarrochi J. Oakland, CA, Context Press, 2013, pp 140–165

Seligman MEP, Rashid T, Parks AC: Positive psychotherapy. Am Psychol 61(8):774–788, 2006 17115810

Sin NL, Lyubomirsky S: Enhancing well-being and alleviating depressive symptoms with positive psychology interventions: a practice-friendly meta-analysis. J Clin Psychol 65(5):467–487, 2009 19301241

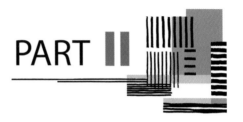

PART II

Medical Care

Section Editor:
Ellen E. Lee, M.D.

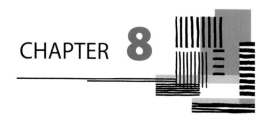

CHAPTER **8**

Diabetes as a Family Illness

A Positive Psychiatry Approach to Diabetes Management

Averria Sirkin Martin, Ph.D., L.M.F.T.

Joana Abed Elahad, M.S.

Ellen E. Lee, M.D.

Editors' Introduction

This case history of a couple, both of whom have diabetes mellitus, describes an effective intervention with medical family therapy. Both husband and wife are supported in learning about the illness, and harnessing and developing their strengths as they approach managing it. They are encouraged to explore their hopes and fears about themselves and their future as they also learn the practical skills necessary to achieve optimum blood sugar control. Ultimately, their commitment to health strengthens their relationship and their connection with their daughter.

SUMMARY

Robert was a 62-year-old Hispanic man who presented at a primary care clinic in San Bernardino County with type 2 diabetes mellitus (T2DM) in hyperosmolar state, including blurred vision, fatigue, rapid breathing, and confusion. Robert was accompanied to this appointment with the primary care provider (PCP) by his spouse, Elizabeth. Robert had been diagnosed with T2DM approximately 10 years earlier, and had been inconsistent in managing his disease and frequently (approximately twice per month) presented at the clinic with complications of his illness. After providing insulin and fluids to treat Robert's acute symptoms, the PCP requested immediate assessment and follow-up by one of us (ASM), the medical family therapist (MedFT) on rotation. The MedFT conducted a brief intake appointment during Robert's primary care visit and then scheduled an initial 30-minute follow-up appointment with the patient and spouse within 1 week.

Diabetes mellitus is an illness that affects a large percentage of the population and has health complications that are unparalleled by other diseases. Both the prevalence and the incidence of T2DM are rising worldwide along with increased obesity rates and westernization of lifestyle (Inzucchi et al. 2013). Concurrently, the number of family members who provide care for their loved one with diabetes continues to grow. Family members play an essential role in the management of diabetes; however, the burden of providing care can be overwhelming and deleterious for the entire family unit (Batty and Fain 2016; Yi et al. 2008). The medical family therapy model conceptualizes illness through overlapping biopsychosocial and systemic lenses. This perspective provides a constructive, strength-based vehicle for supporting individuals and family members impacted by diabetes in navigating the trials and tribulations often associated with their diagnosis. Positive psychological traits such as perceived self-efficacy, optimism, and increased individual and family resilience have been associated with better physical and psychological health outcomes (Martin et al. 2015b). Accordingly, clinical interventions aimed at increasing these positive psychological traits may have positive influence in cases of chronic illnesses. In this chapter, a composite case is presented to illustrate the application of the medical family therapy model to T2DM management.

PERSON

Chief Complaint and Presentation

Robert and Elizabeth were active members in the therapeutic process. Both identified as second-generation Mexican Americans and were bilingual English and Spanish speakers. All appointments were conducted in English. As previously noted, Robert and his spouse were initially introduced to the MedFT during a primary care visit. His PCP referred him to the MedFT due to ongoing complications (i.e., hyperosmolar state, neuropathy) related to his chronic T2DM diagnosis, high health care utilization, and persistent uncontrolled blood sugar. Because of the patient's lethargic state during the primary care visit, the MedFT made only brief contact (10 minutes) during the initial visit to 1) explain the PCP referral, including the process of working with the MedFT and the potential benefits, and 2) schedule a follow-up appointment with the MedFT at the clinic within 1 week. Both patient and spouse were amenable to a course of five weekly visits with the MedFT with the hope of improving the patient's functioning and diabetes management.

It is important to note that behavioral issues such as depression, anxiety, cognitive impairment, and alcohol abuse are often overlooked in primary care settings and are observed in a high percentage of noncompliance cases (Robinson and Reiter 2007). For this reason, at the close of the brief consultation, the MedFT requested that Robert complete a number of routine self-report assessments before his initial medical family therapy appointment. In this case, Robert was given several brief measures to assess his current understanding of diabetes (questionnaires assessing diabetes knowledge [Fitzgerald et al. 1998], diabetes empowerment [Anderson et al. 2000], and diabetes self-efficacy [Lorig et al. 1996]), quality of life (abbreviated World Health Organization Quality of Life questionnaire [WHOQOL-BREF; WHOQOL Group 1998]), optimism (Life Orientation Test—Revised; Scheier et al. 1994), and individual and interpersonal resilience (Multidimensional Individual and Interpersonal Resilience Measure; Martin et al. 2015a). In addition, brief mental health measures were provided in order to assess for depression (Patient Health Questionnaire–2 [PHQ-2] [two-item] screening; Kroenke et al. 2001) and anxiety (Beck Anxiety Inventory; Derogatis and Spencer 1993). The MedFT also screened for alcohol abuse and cognitive impairment during the initial consultation.

Background

In Robert's self-report, the MedFT noted suboptimal diabetes knowledge and low levels of diabetes empowerment and self-efficacy, as well as moderate levels of optimism and individual and interpersonal resilience. In addition, the MedFT noted elevated scores on the PHQ-2 screener for depression, indicating the need for further assessment. Robert scored in the moderately severe depression range on the PHQ-9 (completed in session based on elevated screener). There was no indication of alcohol abuse or cognitive impairment. All results were recorded in the patient chart, and his depression score was directly communicated to the PCP for immediate medical follow-up in tandem with the medical family therapy intervention.

During the initial consultation, the MedFT used motivational interviewing to gain a broad understanding of the history of the illness from the patient's point of view, including life context (home life, family relationships, and activity questions), and functional analysis—problem specification (i.e., diabetes management), hypothesis generation (i.e., what the barriers to success are, what the potential resources are), and identification and teaching of alternative behaviors (to be accomplished in subsequent appointments). Motivational interviewing techniques include reflective listening, open-ended questions, and spotlighting stressors and resources associated with potential behavior change. Motivational interviewing was used throughout therapy to assist the patient in examining the impact of his diabetes on his goals and subsequently as an intervention tool for increasing perceived self-efficacy, optimism, and resilience to support behavior change.

Initially, Robert was hesitant to discuss his T2DM with the MedFT and looked to his wife to act as the voice for the couple. It became immediately evident that Elizabeth was the "family health expert" and would be a key player in the management of Robert's illness. Although Elizabeth expressed concern regarding her husband's diagnosis and frequent trips to primary care, she appeared to minimize the severity of his illness and need for increased care. She made passive comments such as "Robert is taking the necessary medications" and "There isn't much more we can do." Robert appeared aloof, defeated, and disengaged during the initial visit; he noted that he felt incapable of managing his illness and felt that the future was "out of [his] control." This disconnection to the illness in both members underscored the need for nonjudgmental, in-depth, systemic assessment of Robert's diabetes diagnosis, challenges faced by family, and inherent strengths and resources to support better functioning.

History

Over the course of treatment, the MedFT learned that both members of the couple were diagnosed with T2DM. Elizabeth was diagnosed with gestational diabetes when she was pregnant with her daughter but was "not considered diabetic until about 6 years ago." Robert was diagnosed with diabetes about 10 years ago. When Robert was first diagnosed, he was under the impression that he was simply having a problem with his foot. He said that he "felt like [his] sock was bunched up in [his] shoe all the time." He made an appointment with a podiatrist and learned that the cause of his "strange sensation" was neuropathy. The MedFT asked, "What was the first thing that came to mind when you were diagnosed with diabetes?" Robert replied, "Denial." He said that he did not understand how it could have happened, he considered himself a moderately active and healthy man, and diabetes did not run in his family. Elizabeth's experience of discovery was quite different; she said that she was "just waiting for it to happen." Her mother had diabetes, so Elizabeth "knew realistically that one day [she] would have diabetes too." It became evident that this powerless narrative was dictating the family's perception of their diabetes diagnoses, as well as Robert's inconsistent diabetes management. They saw the illness as something that was outside their control and thus did not believe that they could make a significant impact on their disease trajectory.

FORMULATION

Challenges

Both Robert and Elizabeth were taking a variety of medications to control their blood sugar but were not insulin dependent at the point of intervention. Although Elizabeth's diabetes was well managed with her current medication regimen, Robert needed additional support in taking his medication regularly before reevaluation by his PCP. Furthermore, it appeared that Robert's T2DM complications were closely associated with his mental health symptoms; as he became increasingly depressed, his diabetes management and consequential symptoms became uncontrollable. Elizabeth noted feeling "disconnected" from Robert during these times and unable to provide "encouragement" for him.

It is important to note that the family reported high levels of stress. Both members of the couple were part of the workforce, working 50 or more hours per week in low-paying jobs. Although they were reaching retirement age, they did not know if they would have the means to retire in the future, which increased their overall stress level. Robert shared that this caused him a great deal of sadness and anxiety; he felt that as the man of the house, he should be able to provide for his family now and in the future. In addition, the couple noted that their daughter had recently married and left home, which had been an adjustment for them; they both felt a sense of loss in her absence but had not openly communicated this with each other for fear of seeming weak to the other. As part of the intervention, the MedFT discussed with the family that high levels of stress can exacerbate diabetes symptoms and explored potential methods for reducing the family's experience of stress.

Strengths

The focus of medical family therapy is to identify and harness innate individual and family strengths. Accordingly, strengths will be the focus of the interventions described in the following section.

INTERVENTIONS

Medical Family Therapy

Medical family therapy combines biopsychosocial and systemic perspectives to understand the impact of medical illness on the diagnosed individual and the interpersonal effect of the illness on the family (McDaniel et al. 1992, 2004). Although medical family therapy is typically delivered by a MedFT in a primary care clinic, it can be used across medical settings. Approximately

70% of primary care appointments are related to psychosocial issues; thus, a great deal of time and energy in primary care is focused on changing behaviors (e.g., smoking, poor diet, lack of exercise) to sustain health (Robinson and Reiter 2007). MedFTs work as part of a collaborative team including patients, families, health care professionals, and community groups. Although introductions regularly happen during a primary care or hospital visit, MedFTs are trained to work with complex cases over an extended period of time. Using the primary care behavioral health model, the MedFT (often called the "behavioral health consultant") works side by side with PCPs to manage the psychosocial needs of their shared patients during primary care visits. The MedFT then provides abbreviated postvisit therapeutic intervention as needed. Rather than using a deficit-focused model, the MedFT uses a biopsychosocial-spiritual strength-based approach to support family in navigating the illness. Overall, the MedFT's goal is to support the improvement in overall functioning, in contrast to eliminating the illness.

PATIENT AND FAMILY SUPPORT

Typically, a MedFT is in contact with 10–15 primary care patients per day. When further support is needed, the MedFT then provides an additional one to five 30- to 60-minute follow-up visits to provide comprehensive biopsychosocial care (Robinson and Reiter 2007). When patients have chronic conditions, the MedFT may continue to see the patients quarterly for an extended time. After evaluation and treatment, the MedFT makes clear, specific recommendations to the PCP to support the management of the patient's illness. Although the stage of illness is paramount in how the MedFT will interact with the patient and family, therapeutic intervention is generally strength based, drawing on existing family resources and positive psychological traits. In this way, medical family therapy is characteristically a positive intervention.

Utilizing the medical family therapy model, MedFTs view diabetes as a family condition in that family members play a dynamic role in providing support for the management of the illness. Because diabetes commonly occurs in midlife to late life and causes a transitional period, a diabetes diagnosis in one family member often calls for a reorganization of the family (Fisher et al. 1998, 2000, 2001). Positive family influence has a direct impact on metabolic outcomes, highlighting the importance of including the family system in the therapeutic process. In the second Diabetes Attitudes, Wishes, and Needs (DAWN2) study, researchers surveyed 2,057 family members of people with diabetes and noted an increased need for psychosocial support for and involvement of both the diagnosed individual and family members (Kovacs Burns et al. 2013). Almost 52% of respondents felt the impact of diabetes on their lives, noting a negative effect on emotional well-being (44.6%) and depression (11.6%). Overwhelmingly, respondents noted that they did not know how to help their loved ones with diabetes and wanted to be more involved in their care.

Research highlights the significance of family functioning and support for patients living with diabetes and stresses the importance of developing strength-based treatment models that incorporate all members (Batty and Fain 2016; García-Huidobro et al. 2011; White et al. 2007). It is imperative to consider the association between psychosocial and physiological variables, including the potential influence of family, for patients with diabetes. Psychosocial factors, especially family life variables such as family support and family perception, are large contributors to metabolic control in patients with T2DM (García-Huidobro et al. 2011). Functioning of the endocrine and immune systems is affected by interpersonal and social functioning (Olson et al. 2010). Patients who have family members who are supportive have lower levels of stress, better medication compliance, and overall healthier behaviors. In addition, patients with diabetes have a higher likelihood of depression when they feel criticized or live in a hostile environment; depression in individuals with diabetes has effects at the molecular mediator level and corresponds with inflammatory marker changes (Olson et al. 2010). This holistic view of diabetes can support the prevention of debilitating complications that result from high glycosylated hemoglobin (HbA_{1c}) levels and poor diabetes management. Therapy focused on the development of healthy relationships can provide a launching point for biopsychosocial treatment, prevention, and intervention (Yi et al. 2008).

As demonstrated in our case presentation, families who have a loved one diagnosed with T2DM may be overwhelmed with responsibility and bewilderment, and may have difficulty with acceptance. In a qualitative study of 19 patients and family members who were living with diabetes, White et al. (2007) found that family members were much more concerned about their loved ones' diabetes than were the individuals who had the illness. In addition, they discovered that those with diabetes did not realize the impact their illness had on the family until it was discussed openly. Because family members often experience these feelings in different ways, attention to the family unit's integrity and functioning is imperative for increasing family resilience in the face of a T2DM diagnosis.

PSYCHOEDUCATION

Psychoeducation is a core piece of the medical family therapy model. On the basis of Robert's initial assessment, which indicated suboptimal knowledge of diabetes, the MedFT provided information, such as the following, to increase awareness and support management: Diabetes is a disease that directly impacts the endocrine system and causes instability of glucose levels in the blood (Fisher et al. 2000). Approximately 10% of patients diagnosed with diabetes have type 1, caused by a lack of insulin secretion by the pancreas. In contrast, T2DM is caused by a defect in glucose metabolism or insulin production (Fisher et al. 2000). In 2017, an estimated 30.3 million people or 9.4% of the U.S. population had diabetes; 90%–95% of diabetes cases were T2DM (Centers for Disease Control and Prevention 2017). Although anyone can get T2DM, approximately 80% of individuals diagnosed are overweight or obese, so maintaining a healthy weight is an important, and controllable, part of diabetes management. Diabetes is also more prevalent in Hispanic and black populations (Centers for Disease Control and Prevention 2017).

The early warning signs, initial symptoms, and psychosocial impact of T2DM can be different for everyone; consequently, in-depth interviewing is necessary to understand the unique experience of each patient. The American Diabetes Association (2015) suggests that individuals who are diabetic may feel extremely thirsty, hungry, and tired and may urinate frequently. In addition, individuals diagnosed with diabetes heal more slowly than others, experience tingling or numbness in their hands and feet, and have blurry vision. Effective management of T2DM is important because of its association with increased risks of cancer, serious psychiatric illness, cognitive decline, chronic liver disease, accelerated arthritis, and other disabling or deadly conditions. Moreover, T2DM remains a leading cause of cardiovascular disorders, blindness, end-stage renal failure, amputations, and hospitalizations (Inzucchi et al. 2013).

Many elements are central to diabetes management, including medication management and lifestyle interventions (McKibbin et al. 2006, 2010), and help ensure that blood sugar levels and cardiovascular risk factors remain within a specific range to prevent disease progression. (Medication management is outside the scope of this chapter and is managed by the PCP, not the MedFT.) It is important for the MedFT to support the patient and the family in increasing perceived self-efficacy for healthy eating, increased physical activity, foot care, blood glucose testing, and medication adherence.

Interventions to Strengthen Positive Psychological Traits

PERCEIVED SELF-EFFICACY

Perceived self-efficacy is associated with one's confidence in one's ability to overcome life's challenges and stressors, as well as one's ability to attain goals or make meaning of adversity regardless of the various situations encountered (Benzies and Mychasiuk 2009; Bhana and Bachoo 2011; Seccombe 2002). In this case, Robert's and Elizabeth's experiences of living with and understanding diabetes were quite different from each other's. Elizabeth seemed to attribute (possibly artificially) positivity to the illness, a stance that over time had

minimized and silenced Robert's view of the illness and focus on management. Robert subsequently did not feel a need to take action to manage his illness, was habitually focused on past failures (e.g., high blood glucose, trips to
the emergency room), and displayed symptoms of moderate to severe depression, which exacerbated his diabetes symptoms. In addition, Robert repeatedly protested the inconveniences that accompanied his illness, focusing on
the negatives and complaining about the hassle of changing his lifestyle. He
was extremely concerned that he could not eat all of the sweets he once so
readily enjoyed and did not understand "why this was happening to [him]."
This is in line with the work of White et al. (2007), who found that although
individuals and family members would say that diabetes did not necessarily
bother them, it was on their mind constantly and "bothered them a lot."

One goal of intervention with Robert and Elizabeth was to increase perceived self-efficacy by encouraging problem-focused rather than avoidance-
focused coping. Together, the MedFT and family were able to externalize the
diabetes diagnosis and develop clear problem identification. Additionally,
the MedFT helped the couple to modify their adaptive appraisal by supporting their ability to discover potential solutions, positive expectations, and
acceptance of the diagnosis, and subsequently to shift their cognitive appraisal
of the situation to one that they could manage as a unified team (Huber et
al. 2010). Over the course of therapy, the MedFT and family generated solutions through brainstorming and by evaluating potential options for management (i.e., changes in diet, increased physical activity, reductions in stress)
and began to implement the plan one step at a time. As Robert showed success
in each area, his perceived self-efficacy improved. In addition, with Robert taking ownership of the management of his diabetes, there was a significant reduction in the burden and guilt experienced by Elizabeth.

OPTIMISM

Optimism is associated with one's belief systems and positive self-concept
and represents the aptitude to have a positive outlook irrespective of circumstance (Benzies and Mychasiuk 2009; Bhana and Bachoo 2011; Black and
Lobo 2008). Literature has suggested that optimism is positively correlated
with improved self-care and physical health in individuals diagnosed with diabetes (Yi et al. 2008). Furthermore, research has indicated the psychological
benefits of higher levels of optimism: individuals reporting higher levels of
optimism are less reactive to stress (Martin et al. 2015b).

Robert presented with moderate levels of optimism, in combination with
moderate to severe depressive symptoms. In the beginning of therapy, he often ruminated on negative thoughts about his situation and future. In contrast, Elizabeth was highly optimistic and tried to share her positive worldview
with her husband. As Robert's perceived self-efficacy increased, there were

also noticeable shifts in his optimism. Within session, there was a concentration on increasing Robert's internal attributions to his successes. For example, the MedFT spotlighted how tangible outcomes—controlled blood sugar, weight loss, and fewer primary care visits—were related to Robert's ability to manage his illness and a result of his focus on and dedication to health. Elizabeth was supportive through this process and came to each session armed with a list of Robert's successes over the last week to provide evidence in support of this positive narrative. The couple was also asked to write down at least one daily success in a journal at home and discuss it over dinner. The couple reported how this activity brought them closer together over the course of treatment and how they began to feel "like [they] were in this together."

INDIVIDUAL RESILIENCE

Resilience is a comprehensive construct that focuses on an individual's capacity to maintain stability, endure, and recover in light of negative life events (McMurray et al. 2008; Waugh et al. 2008) and can counterbalance physical health disabilities (Jeste et al. 2013). Positive psychological resources appear to have a buffering effect on distress levels related to self-care behaviors and glycemic control in individuals with T2DM. Consequently, ongoing assessment and targeted intervention to increase resilience resources can have a direct impact on self-care behaviors, glycemic control, and the ability to cope with stress (Yi et al. 2008). For example, in a longitudinal study of 111 patients with diabetes, compared with the patients with higher resilience levels, the individuals with low or moderate resilience levels demonstrated higher distress, worsening HbA_{1c} levels, and fewer self-care behaviors (Yi et al. 2008). A study of African American women with T2DM had similar findings, notably a positive relationship between higher levels of resilience and better glycemic control (DeNisco 2011).

Many protective factors that contribute to higher levels of individual resilience are noted in the literature (see Martin et al. 2015a); in Robert's case, perceived self-efficacy, optimism, effective coping, and emotion regulation were all positively impacted during the course of treatment. In the beginning of work with the MedFT, Robert did not recognize his natural ability to overcome his illness and positively re-narrate his illness trajectory. Through thoughtful conversation, motivational interviewing, and the support of his wife, Robert was able to increase his perceived self-efficacy and optimism, which supported more proactive coping with his illness and enhanced emotion regulation.

FAMILY RESILIENCE

Family resilience refers to the family system's ability to adapt, adjust, recover, and strengthen in the face of difficult life events, such as the illness of a family member (Masten and Obradovic 2006; McCubbin et al. 1997; Walsh 2002). This flexibility supports the family in restoring stability and reorganizing following difficult transitions (McCubbin and McCubbin 1996; Walsh 2003). Within the literature a number of protective factors appear to contribute to greater family resilience, such as family communication; belief systems, including spirituality; flexibility; family accord; family time and routines; and social support (Benzies and Mychasiuk 2009; Black and Lobo 2008; McCubbin and McCubbin 1996; Walsh 2002).

Robert and Elizabeth reported having access to a close and connected support network of family and friends, but they frequently worried about utilizing their support network for tangible and emotional support. Together with the MedFT, they developed a plan for reaching out to their kin for support when needed. Although they found the first step difficult, once they reached out to assemble support, they were delighted in how united they felt with this network. In addition, they started to discuss their future with family and friends, including their fears about economic resources and their sadness about their daughter starting her own family and needing them less. In a family session, their daughter shared her concerns about her parents' diagnoses and her strong desire to have them in her life. She stated, "My biggest fear is that they won't be around to watch my kids grow up or that their health will decline rapidly in the upcoming years. I need them here, for me and for my family." The increased emotional expression and communication brought the family closer together, strengthening their family resilience and giving them an amplified sense of connection.

According to family resilience literature, spirituality and religiosity can provide multigenerational stability, as well as purpose, meaning, and a sense of connection to something outside oneself (Walsh 2006, 2009), and therefore should be assessed in session. It is not uncommon for individuals and families to gain strength through their spirituality, which assists with their coping. Some people, however, feel a distancing from God or their beliefs when they are diagnosed. When asked if they had experienced any spiritual or existential issues as a result of their illness, Robert and Elizabeth laughed. Both were practicing Catholics and found solace in their belief system. They did not feel that there was any connection between their spirituality or religious beliefs and their illness. Elizabeth went as far as saying, "God has too much on his plate to worry about my diabetes; it is not his problem, and I do not blame him.…You can put that in your chart." Spirituality and religiosity did join this family with a faith community, which was mobilized to provide additional support (Black and Lobo 2008; Walsh 2006).

Robert and Elizabeth agreed that managing their diabetes was much easier because they shared the diagnosis. The couple verbalized that although their symptoms differed—he has severe neuropathy and vision problems, whereas she has debilitating weakness and weight gain—there was something special in knowing that each really identified with what the other was going through. They laughed and said, "At least we get to swap war stories." When considering possible interventions for families living with diabetes, the therapist might take into consideration the ease that a patient may feel about diabetes management if the person believed that his or her partner or family really understood what the experience of this illness entails.

OUTCOME

Robert's therapy with the MedFT comprised six meetings (one during a primary care visit and five follow-up visits). He and his wife presented as a cohesive couple, both respectful and loving toward each other. This cohesion was seen as one of their greatest strengths and provided a stable foundation for work with the MedFT. Both Robert and Elizabeth lived with a high degree of blame and sadness related to their illness. This was not something that they had the ability to share in the past, as they avoided the subject and thereby allowed Robert's illness to get "out of control." Rather than focusing on deficits and blaming, the MedFT worked with Robert and Elizabeth to identify and harness the couple's strengths to support better coping and management of their illness.

Over the course of treatment, the couple shared that the illness would now only strengthen their marital bond over the years. They both agreed that although diabetes carries a heavy burden, if they "are responsible with food (eat sugar-free everything), medications, and physical activity, it is not a curse. ...It is just [their] job to maintain it." This was an obvious shift from their original narrative. When asked about future coping strategies, they continued to mention that it really was all about management and support.

Even at the end of therapy, the couple continued to verbalize that their biggest concern was what would happen later on as their symptoms progressed and they were unable to be active participants in their daughter's and future grandchildren's lives. They seemed teary eyed as they talked about how the weakness had affected their mobility and how diabetes management includes physical activity, which becomes more and more difficult over time. Sharing this fear with their daughter and one another only strengthened the couple and gave them the motivation they needed to proactively address their illness.

At the conclusion of the medical family therapy intervention, the MedFT shared key points with the PCP and made recommendations to support lasting change. These included 1) continued monitoring of Robert's depression symptoms and current stressors, with referral back to the MedFT as needed;

2) utilizing his spouse as a resource and ally in Robert's diabetes management; 3) reinforcing all efforts toward diabetes management and highlighting Robert's ability to produce change; 4) encouraging ongoing "positivity" journaling by the family; and 5) asking about social support resources and suggesting mobilization of those resources when needed. Although management of Robert's diabetes has made increasing demands on his and Elizabeth's time, they now walk together every day, monitor their blood sugar together, and consult with each other about what foods they should eat for meals. Recognizing their ability to successfully manage their illness was the catalyst for change in this family system.

TAKE-HOME POINTS

- The medical family therapy model views illness through overlapping biopsychosocial and systemic lenses. This perspective provides a constructive, strength-based vehicle for supporting individuals and family members impacted by diabetes in navigating the trials and tribulations often associated with this diagnosis.

- Although behavioral issues such as depression, anxiety, cognitive impairment, and alcohol abuse are observed in a high percentage of individuals with diabetes who are noncompliant with treatment, they are often overlooked in primary care settings.

- Positive family influence has a direct impact on metabolic outcomes. Specifically, functioning of the endocrine and immune systems is affected by interpersonal and social functioning, highlighting the importance of including the family system in the therapeutic process.

- Positive psychological resources appear to have a buffering effect on distress levels related to self-care behaviors and glycemic control in individuals with type 2 diabetes mellitus. Consequently, ongoing assessment and targeted intervention to increase resilience resources may have a direct impact on self-care behaviors, glycemic control, and the ability to cope with stress.

REFERENCES

American Diabetes Association: Diabetes symptoms. June 1, 2015. Available at: http://www.diabetes.org/diabetes-basics/symptoms/. Accessed November 15, 2017.

Anderson RM, Fitzgerald JT, Funnell MM, Marrero DG: Diabetes Empowerment Scale: a measure of psychosocial self-efficacy. Diabetes Care 23(6):739–743. 2000

Batty KE, Fain JA: Factors affecting resilience in families of adults with diabetes. Diabetes Educ 42(3):291–298, 2016 26975301

Benzies K, Mychasiuk R: Fostering family resiliency: a review of the key protective factors. Child Fam Soc Work 14(1):103–114, 2009

Bhana A, Bachoo S: The determinants of family resilience among families in low- and middle-income contexts: a systematic literature review. S Afr J Psychol 41(2):131–139, 2011

Black K, Lobo M: A conceptual review of family resilience factors. J Fam Nurs 14(1):33–55, 2008 18281642

Centers for Disease Control and Prevention: National diabetes statistics report, 2017: estimates of diabetes and its burden in the United States. 2017. Available at: https://www.cdc.gov/diabetes/pdfs/data/statistics/national-diabetes-statistics-report.pdf. Accessed November 15, 2017.

DeNisco S: Exploring the relationship between resilience and diabetes outcomes in African Americans. J Am Acad Nurse Pract 23(11):602–610, 2011 22023232

Derogatis LR, Spencer P: Brief Symptom Inventory: BSI. Upper Saddle River, NJ, Pearson, 1993

Fisher L, Chesla CA, Bartz RJ, et al: The family and type 2 diabetes: a framework for intervention. Diabetes Educ 24(5):599–607, 1998 9830956

Fisher L, Gudmundsdottir M, Gilliss C, et al: Resolving disease management problems in European-American and Latino couples with type 2 diabetes: the effects of ethnicity and patient gender. Fam Process 39(4):403–416, 2000 11143595

Fisher L, Chesla CA, Mullan JT, et al: Contributors to depression in Latino and European-American patients with type 2 diabetes. Diabetes Care 24(10):1751–1757, 2001 11574437

Fitzgerald JT, Funnell MM, Hess GE, et al: The reliability and validity of a brief diabetes knowledge test. Diabetes Care 21(5):706–710, 1998

García-Huidobro D, Bittner M, Brahm P, et al: Family intervention to control type 2 diabetes: a controlled clinical trial. Fam Pract 28(1):4–11, 2011 20817790

Huber CH, Navarro RL, Womble MW, et al: Family resilience and midlife marital satisfaction. Fam J Alex Va 19(2):136–145, 2010

Inzucchi SE, Bergenstal RM, Buse JB, et al: Management of hyperglycemia in type 2 diabetes: a patient-centered approach: position statement of the American Diabetes Association (ADA) and the European Association for the Study of Diabetes (EASD). Diabetes Care 35(6):1364–1379, 2013 22517736

Jeste DV, Savla GN, Thompson WK, et al: Association between older age and more successful aging: critical role of resilience and depression. Am J Psychiatry 170(2):188–196, 2013 23223917

Kovacs Burns K, Nicolucci A, Holt RI, et al; DAWN2 Study Group: Diabetes Attitudes, Wishes and Needs second study (DAWN2™): cross-national benchmarking indicators for family members living with people with diabetes. Diabet Med 30(7):778–788, 2013 23701236

Kroenke K, Spitzer RL, Williams JB: The PHQ-9: validity of a brief depression severity measure. J Gen Intern Med 16(9):606-613, 2001

Lorig K, Stewart A, Ritter P, et al: Outcome Measures for Health Education and Other Health Care Interventions. Thousand Oaks, CA, Sage, 1996

Martin AS, Distelberg B, Palmer BW, et al: Development of a new multidimensional individual and interpersonal resilience measure for older adults. Aging Ment Health 19(1):32–45, 2015a 24787701

Martin AS, Harmell AL, Mausbach BT: Positive psychological traits, in Positive Psychiatry: A Clinical Handbook. Edited by Jeste DV, Palmer BW. Washington, DC, American Psychiatric Association, 2015b, pp 19–44

Masten AS, Obradovic J: Competence and resilience in development. Ann NY Acad Sci 1094(1):13–27, 2006 17347338

McCubbin H, McCubbin MA, Thompson AI, et al: Families under stress: what makes them resilient. J Fam Consum Sci 89:2–11, 1997

McCubbin M, McCubbin H: Resiliency in families: a conceptual model of family adjustment and adaptation in response to stress and crises, in Family Assessment: Resiliency, Coping, and Adaptation: Inventories for Research and Practice. Edited by McCubbin H, Thompson A, McCubbin M. Madison, University of Wisconsin System, 1996, pp 1–64

McDaniel SH, Hepworth J, Doherty WJ: Medical Family Therapy: A Biopsychosocial Approach to Families With Health Problems. New York, Basic Books, 1992

McDaniel SH, Campbell TL, Hepworth J, et al: Family-Oriented Primary Care. New York, Springer, 2004

McKibbin CL, Patterson TL, Norman G, et al: A lifestyle intervention for older schizophrenia patients with diabetes mellitus: a randomized controlled trial. Schizophr Res 86(1–3):36–44, 2006 16842977

McKibbin CL, Golshan S, Griver K, et al: A healthy lifestyle intervention for middle-aged and older schizophrenia patients with diabetes mellitus: a 6-month follow-up analysis. Schizophr Res 121(1–3):203–206, 2010 20434886

McMurray I, Connolly H, Preston-Shoot M, et al: Constructing resilience: social workers' understandings and practice. Health Soc Care Community 16(3):299–309, 2008 18363698

Olson MM, Trevino DB, Islam J, et al: The biopsychosocial milieu of type 2 diabetes: an exploratory study of the impact of social relationships on a chronic inflammatory disease. Int J Psychiatry Med 40(3):289–305, 2010 21166339

Robinson P, Reiter J: Behavioral Consultation and Primary Care. New York, Springer, 2007

Scheier MF, Carver CS, Bridges MW: Distinguishing optimism from neuroticism (and trait anxiety, self-mastery, and self-esteem): a reevaluation of the Life Orientation Test. J Pers Soc Psychol 67:1063–1063, 1994

Seccombe K: "Beating the odds" versus "changing the odds": poverty, resilience, and family policy. J Marriage Fam 64(2):384–394, 2002

Walsh F: A family resilience framework: innovative practice applications. Fam Relat 51(2):130–137, 2002

Walsh F: Family resilience: a framework for clinical practice. Fam Process 42(1):1–18, 2003 12698595

Walsh F: Strengthening Family Resilience, 2nd Edition. New York, Guilford, 2006

Walsh F: Religion, spirituality, and the family: multifaith perspectives, in Spiritual Resources in Family Therapy, 2nd Edition. Edited by Walsh F. New York, Guilford, 2009, pp 3–30

Waugh CE, Fredrickson BL, Taylor SF: Adapting to life's slings and arrows: individual differences in resilience when recovering from an anticipated threat. J Res Pers 42(4):1031–1046, 2008 19649310

White P, Smith SM, O'Dowd T: Living with type 2 diabetes: a family perspective. Diabet Med 24(7):796–801, 2007 17451420

WHOQOL Group: Development of the World Health Organization WHOQOL-BREF quality of life assessment. Psychol Med 28(3):551–558, 1998

Yi JP, Vitaliano PP, Smith RE, et al: The role of resilience on psychological adjustment and physical health in patients with diabetes. Br J Health Psychol 13 (Pt 2):311–325, 2008 17535497

CHAPTER **9**

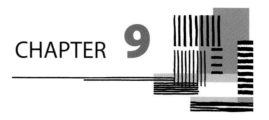

Surfing the Urge to Avoid

Using Acceptance and Commitment Therapy and Cognitively Based Compassion Training to Treat Posttraumatic Stress Disorder

Pollyanna V. Casmar, Ph.D.

Editors' Introduction

This case is striking because a man with long-term entrenched symptoms and dysfunction allows himself to become engaged in a strikingly effective positive psychology–oriented treatment. This is possible because of the superb interpersonal skills and judgment of an experienced therapist who conveys the essential viewpoint of acceptance and commitment therapy. Through a combination of an individualized approach and the application of a manualized treatment, cognitively based compassion training, the therapist helps this traumatized veteran evolve to have a much more deeply satisfying and meaningful life.

The author was a coinvestigator in the Proof of Concept and Feasibility Trial of Compassion Meditation for PTSD, conducted from July 1, 2014, to June 30, 2018 (supported by grant 1R34AT007936-01A1, National Center for Complementary and Alternative Medicine [now National Center for Complementary and Integrative Health]; Lang, Ariel J, PI). The goal of this project is to refine an existing compassion meditation protocol for individuals with PTSD and to examine the safety and feasibility of this approach and to collect data to make initial estimates of efficacy.

Person

R, who had a dark tan and shoulder-length gray hair, was dressed like an aging surfer in flip-flops, cutoffs, and a sleeveless psychedelic T-shirt when I arrived to greet him for an initial mental health interview. I offered my hand and introduced myself. Looking deadpan and straight ahead, he rose stiffly from his chair and shoved the standard Veterans Affairs (VA) assessments for suicide, alcohol use, trauma, and depression at me, with various sections incomplete. He refused my handshake and described himself as "surly" when I asked how he was doing en route to my office. His frustration was because this was the third intake interview he had been scheduled for, each in a different department, and he wanted weekly posttraumatic stress disorder (PTSD) treatment "for a lifetime" as he was 100% service connected for PTSD.[1] Previous notes indicated that he had devised a plan to kill himself for when his dog died or his cancer pain overwhelmed him; however, he had no intention of doing anything about that now. He had "survived Vietnam, so there was no reason to panic." R has given permission for me to use his history for the purposes of acknowledging his significant gains through positive psychology.

He had a chief complaint of ongoing PTSD symptoms, as well as auditory hallucinations due to chronic cocaine use and chronic limiting pain due to prostate cancer. R was disinterested in focusing on his excessive hoarding and organization of ongoing life activities, which took up 40% of his time. He had been coping by drinking 1.5 bottles of wine daily. He had an AUDIT (Alcohol Use Disorders Identification Test) score of 21 (quite excessive), a Patient Health Questionnaire–9 depression score of 10 (moderate), and a PTSD Checklist—Civilian Version trauma score of 63 (moderately severe). Following the interview, R agreed to enter the alcohol and drug treatment program as a condition of entering individual brief therapy with me. To build rapport during the interview, I had used humor to convince him that I could manage his temperament, and I gave direct answers to his questions and complaints. I also explained that the VA placed session limits on therapy interventions because of chronic access issues resulting from an enormous number of veterans of the lengthy conflicts in Iraq and Afghanistan.

A review of R's chart validated that he was a 69-year-old Vietnam veteran with prostate cancer and PTSD from his 2 years in army intelligence as a military police officer. He had recently moved to the San Diego area from rural California. Initially, he presented to the behavioral medicine psychologist

---

[1]The Veterans benefits office had assessed the veteran's files and interviewed him, proving that his behaviors and symptoms were from service. This assessment resulted in a monthly paid service benefit.

from a warm handoff by his primary care physician with vague complaints of being uncomfortable around people except those at the VA. He had previously lived in an open area where he felt safe, and now the city crowds were impacting his anxiety. R was loudly complaining that after having completed 4 years of individual therapy at the Los Angeles VA Medical Center, he had received extremely poor care since moving to San Diego. He referred to vague voices and seeing things that others did not see, admitted to paranoia, and stated that he served Nixon dinner at one of his restaurants. In his meeting with the behavioral medicine psychologist, he said he was involved with organized crime, selling marijuana; mentioned that he had done intelligence work in the military; was evasive about any index trauma; and presented on greeting similarly to the way he had for me, without much humor. His file did not include a Compensation & Pension exam or any notes from his previous therapist. The file included only a history of peripheral neuropathy in both feet, prostate cancer, and alcohol abuse. After this first interview, the behavioral medicine psychologist diagnosed the patient provisionally with schizophrenia spectrum or other psychotic disorder, and ruled out schizotypal personality disorder and PTSD. That psychologist then referred the patient to psychosis specialists at the Center of Recovery Education (CORE), a resiliency-based program for patients with psychosis at the main hospital.

Once R got to CORE, that interviewer documented things more behaviorally, so when I got her file notes, I learned of the no-handshake rule and the convoluted, intellectual, tangential approach that the patient took with her. R was evasive in general and told her that he "feels angry around stupid people, which is about 95% of humans." He also said that he "was furious that I can't just walk in here and get treatment transferred here immediately." After laughing out loud in my office while reading about this interview and prepping for my interview with him, I realized that my positive, realistic approach to patients in the Oceanside Community Based Outpatient Clinic would be a good match for him.

To his interview with CORE, the patient had taken his service connection papers, which documented suspiciousness, sleep impairment (broken-up sleep for a total of 6 hours nightly), anxiety, poor motivation and mood, thoughts of death, inability to establish social relationships, and obsessions and rituals. R explained to the CORE interviewer that he had good interpersonal skills; had planned, before going to Vietnam, to enroll at UCLA, with a long-term goal of becoming a physician; and, on returning from Vietnam, had abandoned this idea because he learned that "people are monsters and he didn't want to help any of them." Because he was unable to distinguish between internal imagination visuals or hallucinated voices, the interviewer from CORE did not diagnose him with psychosis. His symptoms did not meet full criteria for any mood disorder; however, he thought about death a great deal, had experienced depression due to cancer originally, and presented affectively flat with an organized and pragmatic plan for suicide. He had never been hospitalized and had never taken psychotropic medication. The interviewer diagnosed R with major depressive disorder with a rule-out of psychotic features.

In my meetings with R, he revealed his 20-year history of cocaine and speed use. This was in the context of managing and being a co-owner of high-end restaurants in wealthy neighborhoods in Southern California. He had grown up in the Bel-Air neighborhood of Los Angeles, and had known Dean Martin's nephew as a schoolmate, as well as other celebrity children. His parents were married in 1922, had R and his sister, and stayed happily together for 70 years. R says he was a happy, intelligent, and well-socialized child.

Initially an extrovert, R became introverted and a loner after being drafted and serving in Vietnam. However, he was unaware of how much impact the war had had on him because of his intelligent mastery of interpersonal relationships and taking on roles to accomplish a means to an end to do his job in the military. After a marriage of less than 1 year to a woman, he fathered a child. Then he abandoned the infant and mother and simply began working in restaurants, without any remorse or plan. Much later, at age 38, he got married a second time, to an 18-year-old waitress who worked for him. After she gave birth to a daughter and would not get up to feed her as a result of her drug use, R responded to his daughter's cries. He assisted his wife in leaving him and then he raised this child to adulthood. He would appear to an outsider to be a perfect parent who attended his child's soccer games, volunteered at her school, met with her teachers when she was diagnosed with attention-deficit/hyperactivity disorder, and helped her to graduate from college.

However, while raising her, he had to declare bankruptcy because of a poor business investment in a restaurant he co-owned with someone from the Watergate Seven, which is how he met Nixon and his colleagues. After years of working in high-end celebrity-frequented restaurants and using drugs, he began selling drugs and eventually became involved in organized crime. He was growing marijuana and smuggling it across the border from Mexico. Eventually, a 16-person SWAT team tracked him through a business partner whose car had broken down with a million dollars of cash inside, as well as a map to R's home in central California; the authorities had thought R was the ringleader. His attorney managed to get charges reduced, and on the day of his trial, the substitute counselor for the district attorney, who had been suspended for inappropriate behavior, agreed with R's attorney's offer of 30 days' home confinement. R immediately went back to his central California home and grew marijuana and sold it again. He reported that he never touched marijuana and had given up all drug use in his 50s, leaving only his alcohol addiction to tame. Only when he became ill with cancer in his 60s did he stop selling drugs and submit to his daughter's care and "taxi service" to the

Los Angeles VA Medical Center. He moved to San Diego to be near his daughter and 4 months later began treatment with me.

FORMULATION

R numbed his chronic cancer pain and PTSD with alcohol and avoidance of family, as well as other social activities. Because he was no longer leaving his house to earn income, he had little reason to drift from obsessive schedules, foods, and collections of things that kept the rumblings of auditory hallucinations at bay. The more he disconnected, the greater his lack of trust, paranoia, and irritability grew. He entertained himself with his traumatic nightmares, and memories of drug runs, turning them into internalized movies that he attempted to glorify. This was his way of coping with an evil world in which he no longer wanted a part. His disconnection helped him to look dispassionately on his abandonment of his first wife and child immediately after the birth. He thought that this was just the way that he was and lived day by day, leaving unacceptable patterns in his subconscious mind. There was a loss of meaning in his life such that he took a pragmatic approach to suicide. He planned to take his life when the pain overwhelmed him, and he assumed this meant that misery outweighed any enjoyment or contribution he might make.

His resilience, if tapped, was his hidden compassion for others that had been shaped by Vietnam combat experiences. He is an intelligent man who was raised in privilege and enjoyed a celebratory and athletic surfing life outside of his combat years. Overuse of cocaine and alcohol during his years of successful restaurant management contributed to a second unhealthy marriage and left him a single parent. However, his inner loving heart and intelligence caused him to take on this parental role with gusto and tap into meaning again. He had shared with me that he would not commit suicide for nothing. He said that he had survived too much to do that. Also, because he had a daughter to continue to enjoy sharing his life with, as well as other family with whom to reconnect, suicide was not a true option. His thirst for learning and quest for peace left him open to learning about meditation as a method of awareness, coping, and reconnection. Once he began a project and committed himself to it, R intended to complete it. He realized that he had blind spots, carefully chose methods to work on them, and stuck with his choices. Also, he simply craved stimulation and "intelligent" human contact.

INTERVENTIONS

Interventions used with R began with individual acceptance and commitment therapy (ACT). At the VA, this evidence-based treatment for depression is often a secondary choice for trauma intervention because, although many trials have shown significant gains in persons struggling with trauma, research in trauma with this therapy has not reached the VA standard of "critical mass" (Orsillo and Batten 2005). ACT assists with cognitions using mindfulness interventions and commitment to values-based behavioral activation to combat avoidance through meaningful activity. This is in contrast to other therapies that primarily have a symptom reduction focus. ACT uses an informal and personalized approach to care. The therapist assesses the patient's "fusion" to his of her thoughts, feelings, and sensations and assists in providing understanding of the changeability of these while his or her being remains constant as the "context" of these environments. ACT assists with the patient's avoidance of activity and difficulty with finding meaning, by assessing what matters to the patient and by attending to the lack of present-moment focus. Interventions are targeted to increase psychological flexibility (Orsillo and Batten 2005). It was an excellent choice for a patient who craved personalized attention with "an intelligent approach."

After R completed his individual ACT intervention with me, we chose to have him participate in a randomized feasibility trial of group intervention for cognitively based compassion training (CBCT) versus relaxation as a follow-up treatment. The goal was to stretch R's interpersonal skills and expand his interest in meditation or relaxation as an emotion-regulation tool (Casmar et al. 2016). CBCT was originally an eight-session meditation protocol, introduced at Emory University, using Tibetan Buddhist mind training, or Lojong techniques, and showed evidence of improvement in trauma symptoms with breast cancer survivors and children in foster care (Dodds et al. 2015; Pace et al. 2012). In our National Institutes of Health feasibility trial, we randomly assigned traumatized veterans to participate in either relaxation or CBCT; we also refined a workbook, a PowerPoint presentation, and mindfulness homework exercises over three iterations. Revisions were informed by veteran input from qualitative interviews. R was randomly assigned to what had become a 10-session intervention of CBCT.

The standardized meditation tapes in CBCT explain how the mind works, whereas the manualized treatment I developed uses neurobiological, anthropological, and sociological research and modern technologies to teach veterans to take responsibility rather than to blame themselves for normal brain-based activities. CBCT is positive because it assumes patient intelligence and capability of mastery of difficult but relevant concepts. It also allows the patient to understand how to build positive character traits that are already inherent within him or her. It explicitly teaches patients to understand that the similarities between people are great, despite differences in approach, culture, gender, and so forth, and helps to alleviate loneliness while building meaning. The fact that this was a group intervention alleviated R's distrust of diverse participants who demonstrated the concepts being taught. R liked the idea of contributing to science because this was something meaningful he could do to help others. He believed in meditation already; he had meditated as part of his individual ACT treatment. He was willing to learn diverse relaxation techniques if he were to be randomly assigned to that arm of the trial, because anxiety and irritability were primary components of his difficulties.

Because of R's philosophical nature and his distrust of any sniff of phoniness or lack of commitment, a distant therapeutic relationship in which the therapist refused to answer what R perceived as pertinent questions about the therapist would not work well for him. Additionally, because he viewed the filling out of thought revision sheets as insulting, traditional work on depressogenic or trauma-based cognitions in cognitive processing therapy or cognitive-behavioral therapy would not be helpful with him. Repeating traumatic memories and having R work on hierarchical behaviors through prolonged exposure therapy would not have worked because he was already reviewing his memories with some enjoyment. It would have been a fight to assist him in deepening emotion from which he had already detached over the past 45 years. Hierarchical behaviors, again, might be seen as something pedantic.

R and I met weekly for 12 individual ACT sessions, which were immediately followed by 10 group sessions of CBCT.

Acceptance and Commitment Therapy

At the Oceanside Community Based Outpatient Clinic, therapists are provided with bound manuals to assist them in managing sessions for evidence-based care. R was given an ACT manual, which contained homework pages and spaces in which he could record his level of success in completing activities he selected as important and meaningful.

Although R had an issue with being boxed into a manual whose writing he termed "obtuse" and "useless," he agreed that the science of the intervention might be lost if we "threw caution to the wind," so we discussed each lesson in down-to-earth language "translated" by me, with suggestions he made when appropriate. He wrote copious notes in the manual so that he could reference it, should he potentially lose his way in the future.

R objected to the design of the manual and obsessed over any spelling or grammatical errors he found. I used humor with him in relation to his comments because he told me he "liked [his] obsessiveness and [wasn't] willing to work on it." I would thank him for his suggested revisions and accept a certain amount of this argumentative perfectionism, demonstrating my value of his opinions and his natural behavior. If he continued to rail on too long, I might say, for example, "Not everyone enjoys your obsessiveness as much as you do.

Are you ready to move on to the lesson before we run out of time? I mean, it *is* your hour, but is this how you want to spend it?" Then he would laugh with me and return to the content "since [I was] so impatient." Alternatively, we might joke together about how it might take years before the government gave me enough time to revise the manual. This irreverence, frequently used in dialectical behavior therapy with patients who present with therapeutic challenges, builds rapport while also setting limits that eventually become acceptable to the patient. Eventually, R simply mentioned that he had circled some of the inconsistencies to share with me if we had time. At the end of therapy, he offered to rewrite the manual and give it back to me for the clinic to consider based on what he had learned!

We began by looking at the principle of ACT called the "hexaflex," which is the model that largely "sold" the intervention to the patient. R liked the idea that in this treatment one had to accept that life was hard and that a lot of what might be nice to have happen simply was not going to because life was just generally difficult. However, this did not mean that while accepting the difficulty, one could sit around and do nothing. Instead, one was supposed to build psychological flexibility by working on defusing oneself from sticky thoughts, images, and sensations; commit to values-based behaviors to build meaning; and stop avoiding things because of listening to emotions that were neither good nor bad, but instead were simply there. Just because one had a thought or a feeling did not mean one had to listen to it or do anything about it. One of the reasons this avoidance piece was acceptable to R was that it was how he coped with his cocaine-induced psychotic voices: "It is just like some kind of muffled radio playing in the background. At times, I can see it as how I interpret my history and it is kind of interesting and comforting. Most of the time, though, I ignore it because it isn't important."

I explained to R that basically if he were to apply these same meditation principles he had used with the voices to pain, emotion, and images, he would have this technique licked. R explained how he had coped with his nightmares by just allowing them to be there like movies until they played out. Sometimes this impacted his sleep, however, and at other times it allowed him to get back to bed more quickly. We talked about sleep hygiene—getting up to distract oneself in a dark space with boring books or meditating to relax and going back to bed rather than enjoying the full movie. I was careful, however, to congratulate R on his dispassion for the contents of his nightmares. He also explained in great detail how he coped with his pain, since it was not remitting despite "excruciating physical therapy" and yoga. Exercise allowed him to remain relaxed for about half a day, and at times he might take a nap to cope. When he had something to get done, he would complete at least a part of his workout again instead and keep going. I told R that his practicality was fabulous and that I might need to check in on his ability to defuse from mental contents now and again, although we probably could do most of this part of the work by teaching him to meditate. He agreed, and I taught him first the mindfulness of breathing, followed later by present-focused awareness as something he could do daily.

Each ACT session begins with a variety of meditations that "fit" with the lesson of the unit being used with the patient. R enjoyed some of these more than others. The body scan, for example, became a favorite added to his evening schedule to relax and get him to sleep more quickly. This was part of his valued behavioral cluster of maintaining optimal health.

R also took liberties with the assigned homework when he thought it was not challenging him and would request to revise it. We would spend a considerable amount of time ensuring that I thought he had met the requirements of the lesson while being flexible with how he completed it.

This initial flexibility in approach soon resulted in R taking over the structure of the sessions. When I would meet him in the busy, noisy waiting room, I would find him meditating, eyes closed. He would tell me that because he had "been meditating for 30 minutes already," we could use all of our time for other work. He intentionally arrived early to do this, and I congratulated him on it. We talked about how he had begun to use meditation for painful or irritating medical procedures, such as a recent root canal. He was happy to report that present-focused awareness allowed him to relax and notice the dental sensations as what they were; his body could relax and not create the usual neck aches he had experienced during these procedures previously.

R also would explain that he had not done "the homework we made up together." The details of what he had devised instead were much more meaningful and fascinating. After we had spent time in a previous session hammering out what needed to be addressed and brainstorming workable ideas, he would mull over this content and devise something better. We had designed, for example, a long-term goal for him to teach surfing to homeless kids; therefore, he was going to visit some agencies to see what they offered, as a step toward meaningful spiritual growth. He decided instead to go to church! He did this despite "hat[ing] the phoniness of Christianity" because he wanted to see if he could be without judgment during the service, and he had discovered, while looking for ideas on the Internet, that this particular church was involved with teaching surfing to homeless kids. R stated, "I didn't have the patience or energy to come up with a way to help homeless kids on my own. If I can tolerate the service, maybe I could become a part of their surfing team." This is a clear example of how engaging the patient in a process of meaning making ignites internal interest and commitment to change and growth.

The other part of ACT that was especially important to R was that I was willing to be myself during our meetings and share personal stories that made sense given what he was expressing. We talked about how he could not even get out of bed because of depression, and I explained that I had experienced a major depressive episode after a series of four family deaths hit my home in a 6-month period. I told him that some days I thought about what parts of my body were really dirty and had to be washed, so I could look decent for trips out of the house, because I was so exhausted I could not bear to get into the shower. This kind of deep sharing that was authentic allowed R to share his frustrations with his daughter, whom he loved so deeply. He said she could not seem to understand his obsessions and his lack of desire to connect with anyone due to trauma. Our sharing led to a deep processing of what he had tried, and hit on his ongoing sadness about being unable to connect. We engaged in a role-play of how he might try again.

Connecting personally with patients is a hallmark of positive psychology practice, because distance intimates that the patient is under one's care, when in fact the therapist facilitates the patient's care of himself or herself. If therapists are honest, psychiatric work is bidirectional in nature: the patient is inspired to grow as he or she is not isolated in his of her experience, while the practitioner becomes deeply rooted through the resilience discovered in the patient. This resilience compels therapists to continue to search for ways to assist and be present with others while discovering their own goodness. It reminds therapists that they too are resilient when the low points of their own human experience cause them to question their professional interest or commitment to care. Learning manualized treatments at first causes a certain amount of rigid adherence to care that needs to be loosened by remembering how much personal presence adds to protocol. Many times, the mix of relationship to protocol needs to be adjusted to meet the specific needs of the dyad in the room.

By the time we had nearly completed our sessions, R had given up alcohol entirely, reestablished contact with his extended family, and committed to trying surfing again despite neuropathy in his feet that hindered his ability to feel his moves on the board. He was encouraged to attempt small conversations when shopping, dining, or grocery shopping to enlarge his circle. Indeed, he met people of interest to him, a fact that he found surprising and gratifying. He met a cable salesperson, for example, who noticed his T-shirt and began to talk surfing with him. He trusted the man enough to exchange emails and to send him surf sites and historic videos.

When we had only a few sessions left before parting, R demonstrated grief and acknowledged that he had returned to having three drinks of alcohol daily. We discussed that he had meditation and meaningful behavior skills to continue to use. However, the relationship we had formed was one of the inspiring elements of therapy that would be missing for him, and he would need to find others to fill in this gap. We would both miss the humor and growth. R was already lapsing into old behaviors of staying inside a bit more, in addition to drinking, and was having trouble meditating. We talked openly about how he did not feel that our work together had been long enough to allow him to have full confidence in continuing on his own.

I suggested that R try the CBCT randomized trial that would be attended by a group of traumatized veterans from any era and with any trauma. He would either learn relaxation techniques, such as self-massage and progressive muscle relaxation, or enter into the group I was leading, in which he would learn techniques of compassion-based meditation for self and others. Because it was science, R stated he would commit to either intervention. Ultimately, he was randomly assigned to the compassion training group.

Cognitively Based Compassion Training Group

In 10 sessions of CBCT, veterans would increase their practice time with au-diotaped sessions from 5 minutes to at least 15 minutes, while also practic-ing behavioral mindfulness exercises that were scaffolded to assist them in growing interpersonally and reestablishing trust with others.

The CBCT protocol began with breathing meditation, followed by pres-ent-focused awareness training, which for R was old hat. He encouraged other group members, complained about the voice on the recordings and the manual as he had done with ACT before, and took humor from me and the other group members in stride. He began walking 5 miles a day, which was not a part of the CBCT work but indicated his commitment to the values-based work we had done together, and was again mindfully doing tasks and expand-ing his meditation.

At the fourth session, each veteran began the challenge of having to no-tice inner responses to small good and bad things that had happened during the day and share them with another silent veteran. The listening veteran was to see when his or her mindfulness wandered from listening to the other person's story and to notice any urges to comment that had to be silenced. After finishing, each speaker told the group what it was like to be heard in si-lence, and then the listener explained what it was like to listen in silence. R had a startled response to this activity in that he found commonality with his part-ner and did not have any intrusive thoughts. He realized that people could be interesting to him if he paid attention.

R reported at session 5 that meditation was easier than relating to others and that, therefore, meditation was a "trap." He stated that one cannot always be in a quiet space and that when he could not find his own quiet, frustration would arise. While saddened that he felt stuck feeling frustrated, he was in-vigorated as he had some understanding of his own reasons for irritability with others. He knew that he was much more comfortable being alone, and that this class was pushing him outside himself. He joked openly with me about how I had pushed him into this and how I would have to "pay."

At session 6, R admitted to the group that he had been very angry with his primary care physician upstairs just prior to group, yet he surprised himself at being able to breathe, state his case calmly, and excuse himself to come to group. As a result, he remarked that he was glad he actually had some inner space now. He also realized that he was prejudging the doctor and others and that his expectations riled him, causing anxiety and anger before he even connected in the moment.

Outcome

After session 7, R was remaining after class to chat with other group members about his involvement in the California Surf Museum's "China Beach: Surfers, the Vietnam War, and the Healing Power of Wave-Riding" exhibit. He sheepishly admitted that he had offered to manage the project because he had many contacts who might donate items from that era. Additionally, his past experiences with catering would allow him to organize the opening night event seamlessly. When I asked if he was nervous about this, he replied that he was surprised to find that he was not because he had so much in common with other Vietnam veterans. "I can't believe you got me to do this," he said. I assured him that I simply had encouraged him, whereas he had done all of the investigation and work. He "blamed" the experience on me because he would never have even gone to the museum if I had not mentioned it and helped him to understand that he had a place in the lives of others. He asked if I thought he could do it, and I was honest in saying that I was sure he would derive great meaning from it and stick to it because he was committed, yet I worried some about his irritability. He just laughed and said that they would understand that behavior because he was a Vietnam veteran.

I have to say, I nearly cried with a confusion of joy and alarm at hearing about this. It was very important to me that R come through his therapy with a greater list of positives than negatives, and I could do nothing to make that happen. I felt my own influence and impotence concurrently, and because I felt so connected to him, I prayed on my own for his success.

R attended through the final CBCT group session and had again remained alcohol free. In fact, he admitted that he had a single glass of wine with dinner at a gathering for his newfound volunteer group and enjoyed it without needing more or feeling guilty. He did not have another glass of wine later on. His depression had remitted, and his trauma remained present, but there was some relief (by two standard deviations).

R and I met almost 6 months later to discuss his comfort with being the subject of the chapter you are reading. His successes went beyond my expectations. R brought me tickets to the Surf Museum's event. He showed me the

Web site he had created for the museum, and he talked about his interviews with the local news, Department of Defense bigwigs, and PBS, as well as an article about the grand opening that he had helped write for the American Airlines magazine. He had not yet gotten further involved with the homeless children because he was too busy enjoying his buddies at the museum. Anecdotally, he said that because of his perfectionistic attitude about getting things done for the event, they had been throwing darts at his face posted to a bull's-eye that I would see at the museum. He plans to become involved in the Junior Seau Foundation and BRO-AM annual surf camp for children with disabilities. He also intends to remain a volunteer fixture at the museum and, better yet, a fixture in his family at greater levels than before.

This is a story I will not be able to forget because it provides strong evidence in support of positive interventions for veterans who appear to be stuck and angry, bitter and unmoving. In 7 months, these two interventions managed to renew R's world and touch an ever-increasing number of lives with his natural loving kindness.

TAKE-HOME POINTS

- Having a more real, less hierarchical relationship with the patient is one of the most positive interventions.

- Allowing the patient to refine evidence-based protocols within the boundaries of good care leads to better care for the patient.

- The mindfulness movement has allowed psychiatrists to assist patients by seeing that wellness is relative and that perfection does not exist.

- Stepwise individual and group therapy interventions for difficult patients can produce more integrated patients who receive peer feedback.

REFERENCES

Casmar PV, Harrison T, Negi S, et al: CBCT for veterans with PTSD and comorbid conditions, making contemplation behavioral. Poster session presented at the Mind and Life Institute Contemplative Studies Symposium, San Diego, CA, November 10–13, 2016

Dodds SE, Pace TW, Bell ML, et al: Feasibility of cognitively based compassion training (CBCT) for breast cancer survivors: a randomized, wait list controlled pilot study. Support Care Cancer 23(12):3599–3608, 2015 26275769

Orsillo SM, Batten SV: Acceptance and commitment therapy in the treatment of posttraumatic stress disorder behavior. Behav Modif 1(29):95–129, 2005 15557480

Pace T, Negi L, Donaldson-Lavelle B, et al: Cognitively based compassion training reduces peripheral inflammation in adolescents in foster care with high rates of early life adversity. BMC Complement Altern Med 12 (suppl 1):P175, 2012

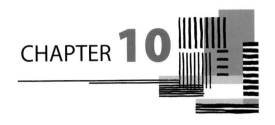

CHAPTER **10**

Use of an Integrated Positive Psychiatry Approach in a Veteran With Tinnitus

Kelsey T. Laird, Ph.D.

J. Greg Serpa, Ph.D.

Helen Lavretsky, M.D., M.S.

Editors' Introduction

This case of a man with several comorbid psychiatric illnesses and tinnitus who engages in a manualized integrated positive psychiatry intervention demonstrates the effectiveness of that treatment and the value of a structured protocol that can be studied and replicated. The case history makes the point that positive psychiatry embraces a variety of treatments that emphasize acceptance, mindfulness, and adaptation to problems using strengths.

PERSON

Jeff was a 43-year-old single black male veteran whose primary care physician referred him to the sleep clinic at the West Los Angeles VA Medical Center. The assessment found that Jeff suffered from sleep-onset insomnia resulting from posttraumatic stress disorder (PTSD) and tinnitus (i.e., sound perception in the absence of an appropriate external auditory source) (McFadden 1982). Jeff reported that his tinnitus developed during his military service over 20 years ago and had been gradually increasing in severity ever since. His attempts to facilitate sleep initiation in the context of tinnitus and PTSD had led to an ever-increasing use of alcohol. As is frequently the case, however, use of alcohol to address a precipitating factor of a sleep disorder resulted in a chronic perpetuating factor for insomnia related to sleep maintenance. Jeff's drinking eventually led to its own set of problems and ultimately resulted in his termination from work. Over a decade later, with several years of sobriety under his belt, Jeff was committed to returning to school to get his bachelor's degree. However, to be successful in school, he knew he would need to improve his sleep. It was at this point that Jeff sought referral to the sleep clinic.

During his intake, Jeff reported that both of his parents had a history of alcohol dependence and were intermittently neglectful and verbally abusive. When Jeff was age 4, his mother was hospitalized for suicidal ideation, his parents separated, and Jeff was placed in foster care with his three siblings. Two years later, his parents reconciled, and Jeff returned to reside with his parents for the remainder of his childhood. After completing high school, Jeff enlisted in the military and served in the army as a cannon crewman for 5 years. Consistent with this job classification, Jeff trained extensively with artillery weapons and reported that this was the primary, but not the only, source of high-decibel exposure. Although Jeff was never exposed to combat, he was a victim of military sexual trauma and subsequently developed PTSD, for which he was recently granted 100% service connection (compensation for a disability incurred through military service). Jeff shared that since the time of his military service, he has occasionally (roughly every few months) experienced brief auditory hallucinations in the form of a male voice saying, "They're going to get you." He denied ever experiencing command hallucinations.

After his honorable discharge from military service due to mental health symptoms (flashbacks, hyperarousal, nightmares), Jeff began working as a security guard, and a few years later enrolled in community college to earn his associate's degree. At this point, he began to notice his tinnitus worsening but did not disclose this to anyone. Jeff had already experienced enacted mental health stigma when he was discharged from the military and feared that if he talked about his tinnitus symptoms, others would think he was "crazy." Jeff began drinking heavily to facilitate sleep. As is frequently the case, the use of alcohol was initially helpful for sleep onset but resulted in difficulties with sleep maintenance, resulting in worsening of insomnia. Eventually, he was terminated from his job as a security guard due to oversleeping and missing several shifts at work. Jeff dropped out of school, became depressed, and began using cocaine, cannabis, and increasing amounts of alcohol in a maladaptive attempt to manage depressive symptoms. When he was unable to pay rent, he was evicted from his apartment. Over the next 15 years, Jeff was intermittently homeless (sleeping in his car, on friends' couches, and on the street), with inconsistent short-term work and heavy substance use.

Three years ago, Jeff noticed blood in his urine and came to the West Los Angeles VA Medical Center for help. He was diagnosed with prostate cancer and subsequently underwent a prostatectomy. Jeff reported that soon after his prostatectomy, he "went into shock" and attempted suicide by taking "all the pills I could find," including a week's worth of oxycodone. He reported that he woke up 2 days later with no apparent medical consequences. Jeff denied ever having had a plan or intent for suicide since that time, citing God and his family (who continued to reside in the Midwest, where Jeff was raised) as protective factors.

Soon afterward, Jeff was admitted to the Domiciliary, a VA residential rehabilitation center, while he underwent radiation therapy. His admission was contingent upon his willingness to remain abstinent from all substances while staying there. Jeff reported that he enjoyed the support from other men at the Domiciliary who shared similar experiences of homelessness and substance abuse. Jeff was able to maintain sobriety for the 5 months that he resided at the Domiciliary and subsequently received a Veterans Affairs Supportive Housing (VASH) voucher. At the time Jeff presented to the sleep clinic, he had been living alone in his VASH apartment for 2 years and had remained abstinent during that time. He had never been married and had no children. He reported that he attended Alcoholics Anonymous meetings regularly and described the other group members, including his sponsor, as "family." He described a good relationship with his siblings, although he saw them infrequently. When asked what his strengths were, Jeff stated, "I'm tough, and I'm committed to my recovery."

At the sleep clinic, Jeff described his sleep as "terrible," stating that most nights he lay in bed for hours before being able to fall asleep. As part of the comprehensive intake evaluation, Jeff was asked whether he was bothered by tinnitus or "ringing in the ears." According to Jeff, this was the first time a health care provider had asked him about tinnitus. He shared with the provider the severity of his symptoms and the major role he saw tinnitus playing in his sleep problems. Jeff had tried everything he could think of, including leaving the television or radio on at night and buying a white noise machine, but nothing seemed to help. At times, he had felt so desperate for sleep that he considered drinking, but he had promised himself that this was not an option. The clinician normalized Jeff's experience by explaining that tinnitus commonly contributes to sleep problems among veterans. Further, the clinician shared that he had recent success referring a patient to a new tinnitus management group offered through the VA Integrative Medicine Clinic and asked Jeff if he was interested in joining. Jeff was eager to try it. He had never met anyone else with tinnitus before, and was excited about the possibility of learning from other veterans.

FORMULATION

Tinnitus is a common and sometimes debilitating symptom with no effective medical treatment. The 12-month prevalence of tinnitus in the United States is roughly 10% (Bhatt et al. 2016). Tinnitus is associated with impaired quality of life (Bauch et al. 2003), depression (Geocze et al. 2013), anxiety (Shargorodsky et al. 2010), and insomnia (Crönlein et al. 2007). In a sample of 182 adults with chronic tinnitus, 76% met criteria for insomnia (Schecklmann et al. 2015). The most common cause of tinnitus is exposure to loud noise. Because most service members are exposed to hazardous levels of noise at some point in their career (Yankaskas 2013), it comes as no surprise that veterans are disproportionately affected. A study of 7,169 nationally representative adults participating in the National Health and Nutrition Examination Survey found that veterans were twice as likely as nonveterans to report tinnitus (Folmer et al. 2011). Tinnitus is currently the most common disability among veterans receiving a new service connection (Veterans Benefits Administration 2016).

INTERVENTIONS

Because tinnitus currently lacks an effective medical treatment, there is a strong need for person-centered approaches that improve well-being and daily functioning, even in the presence of symptoms. Current approaches to tinnitus management focus on helping patients manage their perceptions of tinnitus (using sound) and reactions to tinnitus (using psychotherapy) in order to reduce tinnitus-related distress and disability. Sound-based methods are the treatments most frequently used by audiologists and include tinnitus masking (which uses sound to cover or "mask" the tinnitus; see Schechter and Henry 2002), tinnitus retraining therapy (which uses background sound to reduce contrast between tinnitus and a quiet environment; see Henry et al. 2007), and Neuromonics Tinnitus Treatment (which uses wide-band noise and music to gradually reduce the patient's awareness of and sensitivity to tinnitus; see Davis 2006).

Psychological therapies (Henry and Wilson 2000, 2002) for tinnitus are grounded in a cognitive-behavioral framework, which maintains that thoughts and behaviors cause and perpetuate tinnitus-related distress (McKenna et al. 2014). Research indicates that individuals with tinnitus frequently make negative appraisals about "the unnaturalness of the tinnitus, about it escalating, about it interfering with normal activity, about an inability to cope, and possible psychiatric consequences" (McKenna et al. 2014, p. 3). Such catastrophic thoughts, in turn, often increase autonomic arousal, attention to tinnitus, emotional distress, and avoidance of tinnitus-inducing situations. Avoidance, in turn, is thought to lead to even greater distress (Hesser and Andersson 2009) and disability (Sullivan et al. 1994). Psychological approaches aim to increase awareness of cognitive-behavioral processes and empower patients to mindfully choose more adaptive responses.

Acceptance and Commitment Therapy

Acceptance has been defined as the "adoption of an intentionally open, receptive, and flexible posture with respect to moment-to-moment experience" (Hayes et al. 2013, p. 6). In contrast to resignation or passive tolerance, acceptance is a willingness to experience thoughts, feelings, and physiological sensations in a nonevaluative way. Acceptance changes the function of inner experiences from events to be controlled or avoided to events to be observed with curiosity as a part of living a valued life (Hayes et al. 2013). Initial support for the hypothesis that acceptance reduces distress and improves quality of life for individuals with tinnitus comes from a cross-sectional study of 97 patients with tinnitus (Riedl et al. 2015). In that study, acceptance of tinnitus was significantly correlated with reduced distress, less interference with sleep and other activities, and higher quality of life. Additional evidence comes from a study of 424 patients with chronic tinnitus (Weise et al. 2013); confirmatory factor analysis in that study found good fit of cross-sectional data to the hypothesized model in which tinnitus acceptance mediates the effect of sound perception (i.e., subjective loudness of tinnitus) on tinnitus distress. Furthermore, the indirect effect of tinnitus acceptance on distress was found to be significantly stronger than that of anxiety on distress. The findings from these studies support tinnitus acceptance as a possible target of psychotherapeutic intervention.

Acceptance and commitment therapy (ACT; Hayes et al. 1999) is a cognitive-behavioral therapy that specifically targets experiential avoidance (i.e., avoidance of unwanted internal sensations). ACT has been applied to tinnitus with promising results (Hesser et al. 2012; Westin et al. 2011). A randomized controlled trial (RCT) comparing ACT with tinnitus retraining therapy found that ACT led to greater improvements in tinnitus impact (distress, daily functioning, and catastrophizing) as well as sleep (Westin et al. 2011). Furthermore, tinnitus acceptance at midtreatment significantly mediated the effect of treatment on tinnitus distress posttreatment. Another recent RCT found that 1) decreased suppression of thoughts and feelings related to tinnitus and 2) increased ability to pursue valued activities each mediated the effect of ACT on global tinnitus severity (Hesser et al. 2014). Further evidence supporting the important role of acceptance comes from an RCT of 86 patients comparing the efficacy of relaxation to mindfulness training for tinnitus management (Arif et al. 2017). Mindfulness is distinct from relaxation because it encourages acceptance of internal experience as opposed to change. In that study, individuals randomly assigned to mindfulness training demonstrated significantly greater decreases in distress compared to those assigned to relaxation training (Arif et al. 2017). These studies lend support to the use of ACT and mindfulness-based therapies in tinnitus management.

Integrative Tinnitus Management

The 9-week Integrative Tinnitus Management (ITM) protocol (LeBeau et al., in press) was developed in response to a meta-analysis of 21 RCTs indicating that an integrated approach combining sound-based methods with psychotherapy leads to superior patient outcomes compared to either treatment alone (Wan Suhailah et al. 2015). ITM is an innovative approach that combines education, practical skills, and mind-body interventions in a framework that fosters acceptance and an orientation toward a values-based life. Evidence supporting the efficacy of the ITM program for reducing tinnitus-related distress and depression, increasing mindfulness, and improving daily functioning is presented elsewhere (LeBeau et al., in press).

ITM is provided in a group format. Group therapy is thought to facilitate a sense of universality and hope while reducing shame through corrective emotional experiences (Yalom and Leszcz 2005). Each 90-minute ITM session is facilitated by an interprofessional team consisting of one or two postdoctoral psychology fellows and a psychiatric nurse practitioner. This decision was informed by evidence suggesting that two facilitators are more effective than one (Kivlighan et al. 2012). The nurse practitioner is available to answer specific medical questions (e.g., questions about over-the-counter tinnitus treatments or about prescriptions that may exacerbate tinnitus). In addition, relevant sessions are co-facilitated by a licensed audiologist. A description of topics by session is presented in Table 10–1.

The group is closed, meaning that after session 1, no new members are admitted. Jeff's group comprised 14 members; other iterations have ranged from 5 to 18 members. Content combines components of ACT (psychoeducation about the relationship between external stress, thoughts, feelings, and behaviors; values-based living) with mindfulness practices and teaching as well as audiology-based approaches. An overview of the components is provided below.

TABLE 10–1. Session outline for the Integrative Tinnitus Management program

Session	Topic	Intervention	Practice assignment
0	Orientation and tinnitus psychoeducation	1. Complete pretreatment measures 2. Information regarding causes, symptoms, and treatments for tinnitus provided	None
1	Introduction to mindfulness and creative hopelessness	1. Discuss core concepts of mindfulness practice, followed by a mindfulness exercise 2. Identify ways the participants have been coping with tinnitus symptoms	1. Monitor and log tinnitus experience using mindful awareness skills
2	Control as the problem	1. Begin with a 15-minute body scan with tinnitus awareness cues 2. Identify efforts made to control or get rid of tinnitus symptoms and related negative consequences	1. Begin daily mindfulness practice utilizing MP3 players preloaded with mindfulness exercises
3	Cognitive defusion	1. Assist veterans in recognizing thoughts as internal experiences, as opposed to literal truth or fact via "leaves on a stream" defusion exercise 2. Emphasis placed on the capacity to respond versus react to thoughts	1. Continue daily mindfulness practice 2. Document core thoughts that arise during each mindfulness exercise
4	Sound planning, Part I	1. Begin with a 15-minute mindfulness of present moment sounds, including tinnitus 2. Veterans are educated on how to utilize various external sounds for managing tinnitus symptoms	1. Veterans complete a "Sound Plan Worksheet" in session and test this plan over the next week 2. Continue daily mindfulness practice

TABLE 10–1. Session outline for the Integrative Tinnitus Management program (continued)

Session	Topic	Intervention	Practice assignment
5	Sound planning, Part II	1. Begin with 15-minute mindfulness of sound practice utilizing a sound machine 2. Create a revised "Sound Plan Worksheet" based on previous week's experience and group suggestions	1. Test revised "Sound Plan Worksheet" 2. Continue daily mindfulness practice
6	Valued living	1. Begin with a 15-minute body scan with tinnitus awareness cues 2. Veterans complete the Valued Living Questionnaire, followed by discussion and exploration of personal values.	1. Complete a values exploration worksheet (e.g., "Bull's Eye Worksheet") 2. Continue daily mindfulness practice with MP3 players
7	SMART Goals	1. Begin with a 15-minute mindfulness of breath with tinnitus awareness cues 2. Provide veterans with a concrete tool to assist in setting specific behavioral goals that coincide with previously identified core values (SMART goals)	1. Complete identified SMART Goal and note any obstacles or barriers encountered 2. Continue daily mindfulness practice with MP3 players
8	Course summary	1. Begin with a 15-minute walking meditation (outdoors) with emphasis on using external sounds to better manage tinnitus experience 2. Provide a course summary handout with recommendations for future practice 3. Complete posttreatment measures	N/A

Source. Reproduced with permission from LeBeau RT, Izquierdo C, Culver NC, et al.: "A Pilot Study Examining the Effect of Integrative Tinnitus Management (ITM) on Tinnitus Distress and Depression Symptoms in Veterans." *Psychological Services* (in press). For a copy of the complete Integrative Tinnitus Management manual, please contact J. Greg Serpa, Ph.D., at John.Serpa@va.gov.

Psychoeducation

During the initial orientation session, group members are informed that the purpose of the group is not to eliminate symptoms but rather to teach participants to better manage their tinnitus and reduce the impact of tinnitus on their lives. Information on the stress response and how this response may interact with tinnitus severity is provided. A conceptual framework is presented in which experiential avoidance of tinnitus increases distress. Acceptance, by contrast, is described as a path toward decreased distress and increased engagement in values-based living. Group members are encouraged to reflect on how their own "inner dialogue" (beliefs about tinnitus) has affected physical sensations and emotional responses. As home practice, members are encouraged to monitor their tinnitus severity separately from the extent to which they are emotionally distressed by their tinnitus. The importance of consistent home practice is emphasized, as research suggests that home practice significantly predicts symptom improvement among patients receiving ACT (LeBeau et al. 2013) and mindfulness-based stress reduction (Carmody and Baer 2008). After the orientation, each subsequent session begins with a home practice review to reinforce this point.

Mindfulness

Mindfulness is presented as nonjudgmental awareness of present-moment experience. Mindfulness meditation instructions and facilitation are consistent with previously published guidelines for teaching mindfulness to clinical populations (Wolf and Serpa 2015). Mindfulness teachings and exercises were designed to decrease patients' sense of alienation, encourage self-compassion, and increase perception of their suffering as a part of the shared human condition. Suffering often leads individuals to feel isolated from others, whom they presume to be leading "normal," happy lives (Neff and Germer 2013), and this is particularly true for an internal experience like tinnitus, which can be difficult to describe to someone who has not experienced it. As such, mindfulness is presented as having "an affectionate, compassionate quality…a sense of openhearted, friendly presence and interest" (Kabat-Zinn 2003, p. 145).

Participants are provided with an MP3 player with which to practice daily. Guided meditations included on the audio recording are grounding (5 minutes), mindfulness of breath (15 minutes), loving kindness (10- and 30-minute versions), and body scan (45 minutes). In-session experiential exercises are ordered in a sequence beginning with more basic practices in early sessions (grounding) and followed by intermediate practices (mindfulness of breath, body scan) in later sessions. Because mindfulness of sound may be especially challenging for individuals with tinnitus, this exercise is not introduced until session 4, after participants have had several weeks of mindfulness practice. One purpose of these exercises is to demonstrate that mindfulness can be practiced even in the presence of unwanted tinnitus symptoms. Mindfulness practices can also promote *cognitive defusion,* the awareness that thoughts are not facts but simply mental phenomena that can be noted with gentle awareness and allowed to pass.

Values

Values-based living is presented as a path to a richer, more meaningful and fulfilling life. Psychoeducation on the distinction between values and goals is provided. Values are compared to the directions on a compass; much like north, a value can never be attained. In contrast, goals are presented as concrete "signposts" that can be helpful for marking progress toward a value. Participants are encouraged to identify their core values and consider how they might more actively engage in these values in their everyday lives. Education on SMART goals (Doran 1981) is provided, and facilitators help group members to generate and revise their goals to meet these guidelines.

Audiology

Sound is presented as a method of managing perceptions of and reactions to tinnitus. Several sound types are identified: soothing sounds, which increase relaxation; background sounds, which reduce the contrast between silence and tinnitus (thereby reducing noticeability); and interesting sounds, which draw attention away from the tinnitus. A 3×3 matrix ("sound grid") demonstrates that each of these three sound types can be an environmental sound, music, or speech. Group members generate examples of sounds they judge to fall within each of the nine categories, and choose a sound type they would like to try using in a situation in which their tinnitus is bothersome. Sound sources include CD players, tabletop fountains, radios, electric fans, and anything else that generates sound. As home practice, group members try out the sound plans they have created, which are reviewed and revised in subsequent sessions.

OUTCOME

Jeff arrived early to the first orientation session. Armed with a notebook and a pen, he was eager to learn. Throughout the early sessions, Jeff was consistently engaged with the material and frequently volunteered to share his experiences with the group. After the first in-session guided mindfulness (grounding) practice, Jeff reported feeling "more relaxed" and "at ease." When prompted by the facilitator, he was able to describe the felt sense of these emotions in his body (deeper breathing, less muscle tension, fewer racing thoughts). However, after the first week of home practice, Jeff returned to report that the mindfulness exercises "didn't work" for him at home, such that he had given up listening to the MP3 after just 2 days. Jeff elaborated to say that he just was unable to relax the way he had been able to during in-person group sessions. Again, the facilitator gently prompted Jeff to describe any physical sensations that accompanied this experience. Jeff reported noticing his mind racing; feeling distraction, physical tightness, and frustration; and having thoughts that he was not "doing it right." The facilitators responded with encouragement: "Great! You noticed your experience! That's mindfulness."

It is common for patients to equate mindfulness with relaxation, and it is important for instructors to distinguish the two. Facilitators can begin by saying that although mindfulness practice can sometimes facilitate relaxation, these two concepts are importantly distinct. In contrast to relaxation, mindfulness can be described as "waking up" to one's moment-to-moment experience—even if that means being more aware of unpleasant sensations. If the patient notices that his mind has wandered, his muscles are tense, or his heart is beating more quickly than usual, he is doing the exercise exactly right. Facilitators can normalize and even celebrate the inevitable mind wandering that will occur during mindfulness practice by using the metaphor of lifting weights at the gym: each time the wandering mind is brought back to the focus of the meditation, the "muscle" of attention is strengthened. Continually and nonjudgmentally redirecting the mind to the present moment strengthens the individual's ability to pay attention in the future. Jeff was encouraged by this message and subsequently resumed his home practice.

As the mindfulness practices increased in duration, new challenges arose. In one of the final sessions, Jeff reported that every time he attempted the 45-minute body scan at home, he fell asleep. Again, the facilitators normalized this experience. Indeed, this is a common occurrence, especially in the context of sleep problems. Because Jeff was practicing the body scan before bed, and because he was working so hard to facilitate sleep, he did not view this response as too problematic. He simply began preparing for bed and setting his morning alarm prior to his practice in case he unintentionally fell asleep. For others in the group, strategies were provided to reduce the likelihood of falling asleep during practice: standing or sitting at the edge of the seat rather than lying down, practicing at a time of day when the patient is more alert, and practicing with the eyes open. By contrast, Jeff decided to continue his body scan before bed but to do another shorter mindfulness practice earlier in the day. By the end of the group sessions, his sleep had much improved. He reported that "mindfulness really works!" At the end of the 9-week group, Jeff was committed to continuing and expanding upon his mindfulness practice. The facilitators provided him with resources for other mindfulness and mindful movement courses offered at the VA and in the community in order to facilitate continued practice.

Two months after the group had ended, we followed up with Jeff to see how he was doing. Jeff was still listening to a guided body scan or breath meditation before sleep every night, and he no longer spent hours awake in bed, desperately resisting the ringing. Equally important, he was no longer experiencing urges to resume alcohol use to manage tinnitus-related distress. Jeff had learned to notice the tinnitus, to let it be, and to shift his attention to something else with far less emotional reactivity. Furthermore, he reported that he had reenrolled in community college and that he only needed to take one more class to transfer to a 4-year university. When asked what component of the group had helped him the most, Jeff recalled how seeing the co-facilitators practice mindfulness alongside the patients had increased his confidence in an approach that he might otherwise have doubted. Jeff shared that the single most influential component of the class, however, was the realization that he was not alone. Sharing stories and struggles with the other patients, and learning that he was only one of many individuals suffering from this incurable and often debilitating symptom, helped Jeff to replace his shame with hope. He stated, "Before going to this class, I thought I was weak. I was afraid to talk about the ringing because I thought something was wrong with me. I didn't want to be weird. But after going through the class, it made me realize: I'm tough!"

Jeff's tinnitus was still present but it no longer played a major role in his life. By learning to accept his tinnitus, Jeff was able to more successfully move toward his values of education and wellness. He said, "Some nights, it's more noticeable than others. But I just remind myself that my tinnitus can't hurt me and I use my mindfulness skills. And the more okay I am with it, the better it is."

TAKE-HOME POINTS

- Positive psychiatry approaches incorporating acceptance and values-based living can be helpful even for complex patients with multiple psychiatric disorders.

- A group format can be useful for reducing shame and instilling a sense of universality and hope.

- Integrated multimodal approaches appear most effective for treating tinnitus.

- An interprofessional team providing education, skills, and specific tools within a positive psychiatry framework and group format can be a cost-effective approach for managing a debilitating condition with no simple medical treatment.

REFERENCES

Arif M, Sadlier M, Rajenderkumar D, et al: A randomised controlled study of mindfulness meditation versus relaxation therapy in the management of tinnitus. J Laryngol Otol 131(6):501–507, 2017 28357966

Bauch CD, Lynn SG, Williams DE, et al: Tinnitus impact: three different measurement tools. J Am Acad Audiol 14(4):181–187, 2003 12940702

Bhatt JM, Lin HW, Bhattacharyya N: Prevalence, severity, exposures, and treatment patterns of tinnitus in the United States. JAMA Otolaryngol Head Neck Surg 142(10):959–965, 2016 27441392

Carmody J, Baer RA: Relationships between mindfulness practice and levels of mindfulness, medical and psychological symptoms and well-being in a mindfulness-based stress reduction program. J Behav Med 31(1):23–33, 2008 17899351

Crönlein T, Langguth B, Geisler P, et al: Tinnitus and insomnia. Prog Brain Res 166:227–233, 2007 17956787

Davis PB: Music and the acoustic desensitization protocol for tinnitus, in Tinnitus Treatment: Clinical Protocols. Edited by Tyler RS. New York, Thieme, 2006, pp 146–160

Doran GT: There's a SMART way to write management's goals and objectives. Manage Rev 70(11):35–36, 1981

Folmer RL, McMillan GP, Austin DF, et al: Audiometric thresholds and prevalence of tinnitus among male veterans in the United States: data from the National Health and Nutrition Examination Survey, 1999–2006. J Rehabil Res Dev 48(5):503–516, 2011 21674401

Geocze L, Mucci S, Abranches DC, et al: Systematic review on the evidences of an association between tinnitus and depression. Rev Bras Otorrinolaringol (Engl Ed) 79(1):106–111, 2013 23503916

Hayes SC, Strosahl KD, Wilson KG: Acceptance and Commitment Therapy: An Experiential Approach to Behavior Change. New York, Guilford, 1999

Hayes SC, Levin ME, Plumb-Vilardaga J, et al: Acceptance and commitment therapy and contextual behavioral science: examining the progress of a distinctive model of behavioral and cognitive therapy. Behav Ther 44(2):180–198, 2013 23611068

Henry JA, Trune DR, Robb MJ, et al: Tinnitus Retraining Therapy: Clinical Guidelines. San Diego, CA, Plural, 2007

Henry JL, Wilson PH: The Psychological Management of Chronic Tinnitus: A Cognitive-Behavioral Approach. Boston, MA, Allyn & Bacon, 2000

Henry JL, Wilson PH: Tinnitus: A Self-Management Guide for the Ringing in Your Ears. Boston, MA, Allyn & Bacon, 2002

Hesser H, Andersson G: The role of anxiety sensitivity and behavioral avoidance in tinnitus disability. Int J Audiol 48(5):295–299, 2009 19842804

Hesser H, Gustafsson T, Lundén C, et al: A randomized controlled trial of Internet-delivered cognitive behavior therapy and acceptance and commitment therapy in the treatment of tinnitus. J Consult Clin Psychol 80(4):649–661, 2012 22250855

Hesser H, Westin VZ, Andersson G: Acceptance as a mediator in Internet-delivered acceptance and commitment therapy and cognitive behavior therapy for tinnitus. J Behav Med 37(4):756–767, 2014 23881309

Kabat-Zinn J: Mindfulness-based interventions in context: past, present, and future. Clinical Psychology: Science and Practice 10(2):144–156, 2003

Kivlighan DM Jr, London K, Miles JR: Are two heads better than one? The relationship between number of group leaders and group members, and group climate and group member benefit from therapy. Group Dyn 16(1):1, 2012

LeBeau RT, Davies CD, Culver NC, et al: Homework compliance counts in cognitive-behavioral therapy. Cogn Behav Ther 42(3):171–179, 2013 23419077

LeBeau RT, Izquierdo C, Culver NC, et al: A pilot study examining the effect of integrative tinnitus management (ITM) on tinnitus distress and depression symptoms in veterans. Psychological Services (in press)

McFadden D: Tinnitus: Facts, Theories, and Treatments. Report of Working Group 89. Committee on Hearing, Bioacoustics and Biomechanics. Washington, DC, National Academy Press, 1982

McKenna L, Handscomb L, Hoare DJ, et al: A scientific cognitive-behavioral model of tinnitus: novel conceptualizations of tinnitus distress. Front Neurol 5:196, 2014 25339938

Neff KD, Germer CK: A pilot study and randomized controlled trial of the mindful self-compassion program. J Clin Psychol 69(1):28–44, 2013 23070875

Riedl D, Rumpold G, Schmidt A, et al: The influence of tinnitus acceptance on the quality of life and psychological distress in patients with chronic tinnitus. Noise Health 17(78):374–381, 2015 26356381

Schechter MA, Henry JA: Assessment and treatment of tinnitus patients using a "masking approach." J Am Acad Audiol 13(10):545–558, 2002 12503923

Schecklmann M, Pregler M, Kreuzer PM, et al: Psychophysiological associations between chronic tinnitus and sleep: a cross validation of tinnitus and insomnia questionnaires. Biomed Res Int 2015:461090, 2015 26583109

Shargorodsky J, Curhan GC, Farwell WR: Prevalence and characteristics of tinnitus among US adults. Am J Med 123(8):711–718, 2010 20670725

Sullivan M, Katon W, Russo J, et al: Coping and marital support as correlates of tinnitus disability. Gen Hosp Psychiatry 16(4):259–266, 1994 7926702

Veterans Benefits Administration: Compensation. May 9, 2016. Available at: http://www.benefits.va.gov/REPORTS/abr/ABR-Compensation-FY15-05092016.pdf. Accessed November 16, 2017.

Wan Suhailah WH, Mohd Normani Z, Nik Adilah NO, et al: The effectiveness of psychological interventions among tinnitus sufferers: a review. Med J Malaysia 70(3):188–197, 2015 26248783

Weise C, Kleinstäuber M, Hesser H, et al: Acceptance of tinnitus: validation of the Tinnitus Acceptance Questionnaire. Cogn Behav Ther 42(2):100–115, 2013 23627873

Westin VZ, Schulin M, Hesser H, et al: Acceptance and commitment therapy versus tinnitus retraining therapy in the treatment of tinnitus: a randomised controlled trial. Behav Res Ther 49(11):737–747, 2011 21864830

Wolf C, Serpa JG: A Clinician's Guide to Teaching Mindfulness: The Comprehensive Session-by-Session Program for Mental Health Professionals and Health Care Providers. Oakland, CA, New Harbinger Publications, 2015

Yalom ID, Leszcz M: Theory and Practice of Group Psychotherapy. New York, Basic Books, 2005

Yankaskas K: Prelude: noise-induced tinnitus and hearing loss in the military. Hear Res 295:3–8, 2013 22575206

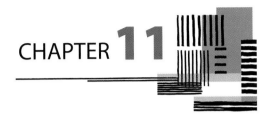

CHAPTER **11**

Building Resilience to Chronic Stress in Dementia Caregivers

Keri Biscoe, M.D.

Dan Li, B.A.

Helen Lavretsky, M.D., M.S.

Editors' Introduction

Rather than focusing on the demoralization, depression, and burn-out that occur with great prevalence among caregivers for individuals with dementia, the positive psychiatry approach seeks to enhance caregivers' wellness within the context of their stressful situations. This case of a woman in her late 60s who is struggling with important decisions regarding her mother's care is striking because of the degree of change she was able to make with an uncomplicated intervention in which she could engage at home.

SUMMARY

Natalie is a 67-year-old woman who was experiencing severe stress from being the primary caretaker for her mother, a 90-year-old who suffers from dementia. Natalie's stress was so severe that she was prescribed lorazepam and clonidine for anxiety and comorbid high blood pressure. After her mother had a fall that resulted in hospitalization, Natalie's anxiety worsened. We prescribed Natalie four interventions: Kirtan Kriya yoga, strength building, savoring, and Coherent Breathing, all aimed to reduce her anxiety and blood pressure. One month after starting the intervention, Natalie scored better on scales of anxiety, depressed mood, positive well-being, self-control, and general health. She has decreased her lorazepam dosage and plans to eventually discontinue anxiolytic medications altogether, under the supervision of her primary care physician.

PERSON

Natalie is a 67-year-old aesthetician whose 90-year-old mother suffers from Alzheimer's disease (AD). My (KB) first encounter with Natalie occurred when she brought her mother to my ophthalmology office for cataract evaluation. Despite her cataracts, Natalie's mother maintained good vision, so we decided not to pursue surgery but rather to follow up every 6 months. One year later, the mother's cataracts were stable, but it was clear that her dementia was worsening. Natalie looked worn and had lost weight. She admitted that she was struggling to take care of her mother. She stated that the physical demands of caregiving, coupled with responding to her mother's behavioral problems, were taking a toll on her and her marriage. She was considering moving her mother to an assisted living facility because the stress of caregiving was overwhelming her, yet making this decision added to her stress. She confided in me that normally she did not speak about "these things" for fear of what others might think. "I appreciate you as a doctor taking the time to talk to me about this."

In addition to being a practicing ophthalmologist, I have always had an interest in psychosocial issues. As residents of a small rural community, Natalie and I spoke socially on several occasions outside of my office, after her mother's follow-up visit. During this time I was engaged in a curriculum and attending seminars that taught techniques that are fundamental to positive psychiatry. Because of the rapport that Natalie and I had established, we were both willing to explore strategies that I had been learning for dealing with stress —strategies that might help Natalie.

Natalie is a slender woman who owns her own business and is in a stable marriage with grown children who are doing well. She normally maintains a good diet and exercises. She has no prior psychiatric diagnoses. Except for what she describes as "a bout of postpartum depression" after one of her children was born, she enjoyed a physically and emotionally healthy life until the stress of caring for her mother became overwhelming, particularly over the past year since her mother came to live with Natalie and her husband. She stated that she often felt anxious, had trouble sleeping at night, and had experienced several panic attacks. She said, "When I stepped on the scale and saw how much weight I have lost, I burst into tears." Her internist started her on lorazepam 1.0 mg daily and a clonidine transdermal patch, because Natalie had been diagnosed with high blood pressure in recent months. The fact that she was placed on medication exacerbated Natalie's anxiety. She felt she needed to "take control" of herself and get off the medications as soon as possible.

During conversations spanning several months, I learned that Natalie's mother was hospitalized due to a fall at home. Natalie felt guilty about the fall, blamed herself, and ruminated about how she could have done things differently to prevent it. The fact that her mother was now being cared for by hospital staff had little effect on Natalie's anxiety. She relayed that her panic symptoms tended to flare as she drove to the hospital to visit her mother. Also, although her mother had never been aggressive toward her daughter, Natalie was getting reports of her mother biting the nurses and showing aggressive behavior in the hospital.

FORMULATION

As the age of the United States population increases, AD and other age-related dementias are affecting more and more households. Currently, over 5 million Americans have a diagnosis of AD. The prevalence of AD is expected to increase by 29% by the year 2025 and nearly 300% by 2050, at which time 13.8 million Americans are expected to have the disease (Alzheimer's Association 2018).

During the next decade, the number of relatives and loved ones who provide informal caregiving will also continue to rise. The toll this takes on loved ones—emotionally, physically, and financially—is staggering. The effects are felt within the family structure and at the workplace. In 2017, approximately 16 million unpaid caregivers provided 18.4 billion hours of care, valued at $230.1 billion (Alzheimer's Association 2018). AD has been reported to cost U.S. businesses $61 billion annually; 50% of this cost is due to lost productivity and replacement of workers who become family caregivers. Not included in this number are the direct financial costs to family caregivers or the costs associated with depression among family members providing care.

The personal, social, and health impacts of dementia caregiving have been well documented in recent years. Because of the unique and extreme challenges associated with caring for someone with cognitive and behavioral impairment, family members are being asked to perform complex tasks similar to those carried out by paid health care providers. Thirty-eight percent of family caregivers, the majority of whom are over age 65, have been providing often constant care for more than 5 years. These caregivers are likely to report high levels of physical, emotional, and financial distress as a direct result of caregiving responsibilities (Wolff et al. 2016). They are more likely to report family conflict, spend less time with other family members, and give up vacations, hobbies, and other personal activities. Increased caregiver burden and depression are related to the level of patient disability and behavioral problems.

In the last months of a patient's life, 40%–50% of caregivers have symptoms that meet the criteria for clinical depression (Lavretsky 2005). There are a number of factors that make providing care for a patient with AD emotionally draining and difficult. Because these patients live for an average of 8 years after the initial diagnosis and may live for as long as 20 years after the onset of symptoms, the duration of the period of caregiving is exceptionally long and especially challenging. As a result of the loved one's deterioration in mental ability and functioning, caregiver grieving and depression may start before the death of the patient and may persist following the patient's death, leading to the development of chronic and recurrent depression. Other risk factors for caregiver depression include female gender, prior history of depression, poor health, low income, and family conflict (Covinsky et al. 2003).

Natalie stated that her ongoing struggle with anxiety was causing her to feel frustrated with herself and depressed. During our conversations, while listening to her words and observing her nonverbal body language, I thought of how to apply principles of positive psychiatry. To enhance her sense of well-being, I employed techniques such as strength spotting, prizing, reframing, modeling compassion, and building on what was already strong in Natalie. For most of her life, she had been a woman whose self-efficacy provided her with a measure of economic and intellectual independence, enhancing her quality of life. As a successful small business owner, she demonstrated a strong work ethic, and the nature of her business gave her a platform to express her creativity. Natalie was a weekly churchgoer, and her faith in the Divine was a source of great comfort and support for her. She also enjoyed the social support of fellow churchgoers, her family, and her friends. She occasionally walked for exercise and maintained a healthy diet.

One of the challenges to Natalie's well-being was her lack of time for herself. Although her four children were successful adults running their own households, the demands on Natalie to take care of her household, her marriage, her mother, and her business left little time for self-care. There were several cultural challenges as well. In early conversations, Natalie was wary of being stigmatized as "crazy" because she was struggling with anxiety. She engaged in negative self-talk, telling herself to "get past this already" and "pull yourself together" when her anxiety caused her to feel out of control. Her marriage, while long-lasting, posed its own challenges. Like many women, Natalie often found herself prioritizing the wishes and needs of others before her own. In response to marital tension, she started expressing herself and her feelings less and less, opting to go along with her husband's wishes in order to "keep the peace." Worry about financial matters posed another challenge. Her business had been slowing down for some time, and she and her husband were experiencing friction about whether to move to a less expensive home. A related challenge was insomnia. She stated that she had trouble falling asleep because "my mind is always working." Part of what kept her awake was the dilemma of what to do when her mother was released from the hospital.

INTERVENTIONS

One of the first approaches I used to support Natalie was to normalize her anxiety as a natural response to several major life stressors she was experiencing: marital discord, an uncertain financial future, the possibility of relocating, and illness in the family. I explained how common it is for the loved ones of patients with AD to become particularly overwhelmed in the caregiving role, and that the toll this was taking on her own health and her marriage was a concern that could be addressed. She was clearly relieved to learn how common anxiety is and that she was "not crazy" and "not alone." When I pointed out that our culture generally does not teach us how to constructively manage anxiety, fear, or other emotions that are difficult to feel and therefore it is small wonder that so many people struggle at some time in their lives, she saw how she could be more compassionate with her self-talk as she moved through this experience. I reflected to her that her "can do" attitude and determination to stop taking medication were strengths she could use to help motivate her to practice self-care techniques that may help restore her sense of well-being. She said she was willing to try self-care techniques, with the hope of substituting these for taking medication.

Given her particular challenges and strengths, I chose the following four interventions for Natalie to practice: Kirtan Kriya yoga, strength building, savoring, and Coherent Breathing. I chose these interventions for several reasons.

As a caregiver, wife, and business owner, Natalie did not have much time in her schedule that was for her. Kirtan Kriya is a 12-minute yoga practice that has been studied for caregiver stress and has been proven to address several of Natalie's concerns, including reducing anxiety and improving sleep. Lavretsky et al. (2013) demonstrated that when stressed caregivers gave themselves 12 minutes daily for a Kirtan Kriya practice for 8 weeks, the benefits included improved mental health, depression, anxiety, and sleep; a reduction in inflammation and cellular aging; and brain fitness effects, with improved cognitive and executive functioning (Lavretsky et al. 2013; Pomykala et al. 2012). The Kirtan Kriya group also showed reduction in an array of biochemical stress markers, as well as an increase in telomerase, an enzyme that is thought to play a role in slowing the aging process (Black et al. 2013). After 8 weeks of daily 12-minute Kirtan Kriya yoga practice, study participants reported a generally enhanced sense of well-being and sense of control over their lives. Perhaps Natalie could benefit from Kirtan Kriya in ways similar to those of the participants in these studies.

By setting an intention to act on a character strength in an enjoyable way, this positive reframing would allow Natalie to focus on her strengths (rather than weaknesses) and to become mindful of doing something that she enjoys every day. Research by Seligman et al. (2005) has shown that participants who were asked to use their strengths in novel and creative ways showed increased happiness and decreased depression scores.

Similarly, writing three good things that happened each day and savoring them would help to seat her attention in what brings her energy and joy and gratitude. I imagined that finding things to appreciate might come naturally to Natalie given her occupation as an aesthetician. This practice has also been shown by Seligman et al. (2005) to be effective in promoting well-being.

The positive intervention of Coherent Breathing has a plethora of benefits and applications due to the effects of rebalancing the autonomic nervous system. This has been elucidated by extensive basic science and clinical research. As stated by Brown and Gerbarg (2012), who have published extensively on the subject, Coherent Breathing is "gentle breathing at 4.5–6.0 breaths per minute, with equal inhalation and exhalation, in and out through the nose with no force or pressure." The Coherent Breathing 2 Bells recording that I prescribed for Natalie allows her to pace her breathing to 5 breaths per minute by simply following the chimes of two different bells, which guide the timing of inhalation and exhalation (www.coherence.com). This slowed breathing activates the parasympathetic nervous system, which creates a cascade of positive, restorative effects on emotion regulation as well as on the cardiovascular, gastrointestinal, metabolic, and cerebrovascular systems (Streeter et al. 2012). I chose this positive intervention to assist Natalie with her anxiety because it has been proven effective in multiple clinical populations, including those with posttraumatic stress disorder and generalized anxiety disorder. Additionally, with the proven benefit of lowering blood pressure, Coherent Breathing might help Natalie reach her goal of discontinuing her anxiolytic and antihypertensive medications. This evening practice could also facilitate her falling asleep at night.

I also selected these four interventions because they are portable and do not take much time to complete. When Natalie's busy schedule includes travel, these interventions are sustainable because they take less than 30 minutes of her morning and less than 30 minutes of her evening.

Before prescribing these positive psychiatry techniques, I asked Natalie to fill out the Psychological General Well-Being Index (PGWBI; Lundgren-Nilsson et al. 2013), which is a 22-item questionnaire that scores six dimensions (Anxiety, Depressed Mood, Positive Well-Being, Self-Control, General Health, and Vitality) to assess quality of life. Higher scores reflect a better quality of life. Natalie completed the questionnaire referencing how she felt during the preceding 2 weeks. Her PGWBI score was 73. I then prescribed for Natalie specific mind-body practices (Figure 11–1), and we agreed to meet 2 weeks later to assess her progress.

Outcome

The next time we met, within a month, Natalie said she was doing much better. She described herself as being 90% back to how she was prior to becoming plagued by stress and anxiety. She stated that the Coherent Breathing practices had a calming effect, with reduction in blood pressure, and that savoring three good things that happened each day was very helpful "to get your mind to focus on the positive and not the negative." She was surprised that the Kirtan Kriya was the technique she practiced most consistently and was the most effective in reducing her anxiety, in spite of the fact that she had trouble visualizing a column of light coming in through the top of her head and out at the point between her eyebrows. Because of her religious beliefs, the part of the Kirtan Kriya practice described as "chanting" initially presented an obstacle for her. She overcame that obstacle by telling me, "I am a Christian woman so I do not chant—but I did sing the mantra." Because I put a YouTube link that illustrates the practice on her cell phone (see Figure 11–1), she found it easy to maintain her Kirtan Kriya practice while traveling.

I listened to Natalie and then reflected back to her some of her inner resources she was using to her benefit, and acknowledged her for the proactive self-care steps she had taken. These positive interventions reduced her feelings of distress and anxiety and empowered her to take several significant steps toward healing herself.

Since our last visit, Natalie had done the following:

1. Made peace with moving her mother to an assisted living facility
2. Moved to a new home that felt more comfortable to her and her husband
3. Been more mindful of putting herself first and not doing everything her husband wanted
4. Been more expressive with her emotions—allowing herself to speak up or cry rather than "bottle it in"

Morning

1. *Kirtan Kriya* (12 minutes): The standard practice includes repetitive finger movements (or mudras), as well as chanting of the mantra "Saa, Taa, Naa, Maa," meaning "Birth, Life, Death, Rebirth," first chanted aloud, then in a whisper,
and then silently for a total of 11 minutes, followed by a final 1 minute of deep breathing relaxation accompanied by the visualization of light (http://www.alzheimersprevention.org/research/12-minute-memory-exercise/; https://www.3ho.org/files/pdfs/KirtanKriya.pdf). A YouTube link (https://www.youtube.com/watch?v=2l9_rCpir_wandlist=RD2l9_rCpir_w) can facilitate Kirtan Kriya practice.

2. *Strength Building:* Choose one of the character strengths (from the VIA Institute on Character) listed below that you identify with. Set an intention of how you will use one of these strengths today, in a way that you will enjoy.

Character Strengths

Appreciation of beauty and excellence	Kindness
	Leadership
Bravery	Love
Creativity	Love of learning
Curiosity	Perseverance
Fairness	Perspective
Forgiveness	Prudence
Gratitude	Self-regulation
Honesty	Social intelligence
Hope	Spirituality
Humility	Teamwork
Humor	Zest
Judgment	

Evening

1. *Savoring:* Write three good things that happened today (big or small) and savor them. Write three descriptive sentences about each.

2. *Coherent Breathing:* Use the 5-breaths-per-minute pattern (using Two Bells recording) for 12 minutes.

FIGURE 11–1.   Intervention instructions for Natalie's mind-body practice.

5. Committed to a daily practice of prayer, especially before going to sleep
6. Found that her adult daughter and her elderly mother supported her decision to take care of herself and not always cater to her husband's wishes to the detriment of her well-being

Of the steps Natalie had taken, she said the most impactful were her daily prayer and deciding to relocate to more affordable housing and to move her mother to assisted living. Her PGWBI scores increased in Anxiety, Depressed Mood, Positive Well-Being, Self-Control, and General Health, and her Vitality score stayed the same. Although Natalie was grateful that her anxiety symptoms had decreased and that she was now using only 0.5 mg of lorazepam to sleep at night, she was still wearing her clonidine patch. Experiencing the progress she had made gave her the confidence to say, "I can get off these meds." She stated it was only a matter of time. I encouraged her to continue the practices and then consult with her internist.

In conclusion, after a brief period of time, the improved self-care approaches to stress management and gratitude practice used in this case had a significant positive impact on Natalie's symptoms and general well-being. When I asked her what she would like to say to health care professionals after receiving treatment for months for her anxiety, Natalie said, "I would want doctors to realize that there are ways to deal with anxiety. I wish they would've shown me first how to deal with it in ways like diet, exercise, breathing—what we've done here—instead of pushing medication first. If I had been shown how to deal with it in other ways, I definitely would not have been taking all these medications."

Natalie represents many patients who want to be able to cope with stress without using medications. One of the take-home points of Natalie's case is that positive psychiatry techniques provide low-cost tools to empower patients to take an active role in cultivating their well-being. This case provides a model for establishing partnerships between patients and physicians and empowering patients to take control over their health and lives. Another important point emphasizes the importance for physicians to explore patients' individual preferences for care. A brief assessment of spiritual or cultural preferences can help shape treatment plans that are meaningful and easy to follow for individual patients. As health care costs continue to rise, mind-body techniques are low-cost and evidence-based approaches for stress reduction.

With rapidly increasing numbers of family dementia caregivers with chronic stress, mind-body therapies can provide powerful tools for self-care and stress reduction. Yoga, meditation, tai chi, and other mind-body practices have been shown to reduce symptoms of depression, anxiety, insomnia, and other symptoms of chronic stress. One pilot study showed that Inner Resources, a six-session yoga-meditation program, reduced caregiver anxiety and depression while improving perception of self-efficacy and emotional well-being (Waelde et al. 2004). Lavretsky et al. (2013) compared the effects of daily Kirtan Kriya meditation with music listening (control) in 49 subjects. The meditation group showed significantly greater improvement in depression severity and overall mental health, as well as improved cognition. Additionally, subjects in the meditation group had increased telomerase activity, suggesting that the meditation may have decreased cellular aging in caregivers. In separate publications of the same study and other subsequent studies, we documented neuroplastic effects on the brain connectivity and metabolism associated with improved cognitive functioning (Acevedo et al. 2016; Jain et al. 2014; Pomykala et al. 2012). Innes et al. (2012) also conducted a pilot study of a Kirtan Kriya meditation program in caregiver dyads. The dyads who completed the 8-week, 12-minute-per-day program reported reduced stress, reduced blood pressure, and improved sleep, mood, and memory. It is unclear how meditation training for caregiver dyads compared with training for caregivers only. However, 9 of 10 participants who finished the program reported that they enjoyed the meditation.

Additionally, Oken et al. (2010) demonstrated that mindfulness-based cognitive therapy, completed over six weekly 90-minute sessions and practiced at home, decreased stress more than having respite periods of equal duration. This relationship held in both test groups examined by the researchers. However, salivary cortisol and sleep quality were unchanged for both groups (Oken et al. 2010).

Whereas most measures of caregiver stress and mental or physical health include subjective or objective questionnaires, direct measures of stress utilize measures of hormonal levels and cellular immunity as physiological indicators of the impact of stress on caregiver health. Chronic caregiver stress has been associated with alterations in both endocrine and immune function. Elderly caregivers are especially susceptible due to a natural waning of their immune systems, the so-called immune senescence, which can be compounded by the effect of stress. Stress hormones are immediately responsive to central nervous system arousal related to caregiver distress. Periods of stress are accompanied by increased activation of the hypothalamic-pituitary-adrenal (HPA) axis and increased production of cortisol in particular. Conversely, dehydroepiandrosterone (DHEA), another hormone product of the HPA axis, represents the body's natural antagonist of glucocorticoids, such as cortisol, and has been inversely associated with stress. Stress hormones are elevated in major depressive illness, and the diurnal rhythm is distorted. Evening levels of cortisol, which are normally low, are increased in patients with depression. Additionally, the stress hormone axis in major depression is resistant to suppression by the synthetic glucocorticoid dexamethasone. Treatment with antidepressants or psychosocial intervention leading to improvement in depression is likely to improve regulation of stress hormones and immunity and have neuroprotective qualities, which will be important for the development of preventive strategies for depression (Lavretsky et al. 2010).

Given the magnitude of the problem of caregiver burden, and the variety of caregiver interventions studied to address it, it is surprising that a number of psychosocial intervention studies have consistently failed to document positive outcomes. However, several randomized clinical trials have shown that interventions that combine a number of different approaches are successful in reducing caregiver burden and delaying time to nursing home admission (Beinart et al. 2012). Facilitating stress reduction in the family caregiver may prove a tangible and cost-effective way to ensure that both patients and caregivers have the best possible quality of life. The early identification of individual risk factors for depression and the availability of preventive intervention can improve functioning of caregivers and delay nursing home placement of patients with AD; improve adaptation to bereavement following the death of the patient; and prevent chronicity of depression. Mind-body interventions lend themselves to stress reduction in chronically stressed caregivers, as well as prevention of depression and other mental and physical disorders, potentially reducing mortality in this high-risk population.

TAKE-HOME POINTS

- There is a demand for integrative and positive psychiatry techniques from patients who want to be less medicated.

- Positive psychiatry techniques provide low-cost tools to empower patients and caregivers to take an active role in cultivating their well-being.

- Mind-body techniques are low-cost and evidence-based treatments for caregiver stress and burden.

REFERENCES

Acevedo BP, Pospos S, Lavretsky H: The neural mechanisms of meditative practices: novel approaches for healthy aging. Curr Behav Neurosci Rep 3(4):328–339, 2016 27909646

Alzheimer's Association: 2018 Alzheimer's disease facts and figures. Alzheimers Dement 14(3):367–429, 2018

Beinart N, Weinman J, Wade D, Brady R: Caregiver burden and psychoeducational interventions in Alzheimer's disease: a review. Dement Geriatr Cogn Dis Extra 2(1):638-648, 2012 23341829

Black DS, Cole SW, Irwin MR, et al: Yogic meditation reverses NF-κB and IRF-related transcriptome dynamics in leukocytes of family dementia caregivers in a randomized controlled trial. Psychoneuroendocrinology 38(3):348–355, 2013 22795617

Brown R, Gerbarg P: The Healing Power of the Breath: Simple Techniques to Reduce Stress and Anxiety, Enhance Concentration, and Balance Your Emotions. Boulder, CO, Shambhala Publications, 2012

Covinsky KE, Newcomer R, Fox P, et al: Patient and caregiver characteristics associated with depression in caregivers of patients with dementia. J Gen Intern Med 18(12):1006–1014, 2003 14687259

Innes KE, Selfe TK, Brown CJ, et al: The effects of meditation on perceived stress and related indices of psychological status and sympathetic activation in persons with Alzheimer's disease and their caregivers: a pilot study. Evid Based Complement Alternat Med 2012:927509, 2012, 22454689

Jain FA, Nazarian N, Lavretsky H: Feasibility of central meditation and imagery therapy for dementia caregivers. Int J Geriatr Psychiatry 29(8):870–876, 2014 24477920

Lavretsky H: Stress and depression in informal family caregivers of patients with Alzheimer's disease. Aging Health 1(1):117–133, 2005

Lavretsky H, Siddarth P, Irwin MR: Improving depression and enhancing resilience in family dementia caregivers: a pilot randomized placebo-controlled trial of escitalopram. Am J Geriatr Psychiatry 18(2):154–162, 2010 20104071

Lavretsky H, Epel ES, Siddarth P, et al: A pilot study of yogic meditation for family dementia caregivers with depressive symptoms: effects on mental health, cognition, and telomerase activity. Int J Geriatr Psychiatry 28(1):57–65, 2013 22407663

Lundgren-Nilsson A, Jonsdottir IH, Ahlborg G Jr, Tennant A: Construct validity of the psychological general well being index (PGWBI) in a sample of patients undergoing treatment for stress-related exhaustion: a Rasch analysis. Health Qual Life Outcomes 11:2, January 7, 2013 23295151

Oken BS, Fonareva I, Haas M, et al: Pilot controlled trial of mindfulness meditation and education for dementia caregivers. J Altern Complement Med 16(10):1031–1038, 2010

Pomykala KL, Silverman DH, Geist CL, et al: A pilot study of the effects of meditation on regional brain metabolism in distressed dementia caregivers. Aging Health 8(5):509–516, 2012 23378856

Seligman ME, Steen TA, Park N, Peterson C: Positive psychology progress: empirical validation of interventions. Am Psychol 60(5):410–421, 2005

Streeter CC, Gerbarg PL, Saper RB, et al: Effects of yoga on the autonomic nervous system, gamma-aminobutyric-acid, and allostasis in epilepsy, depression, and post-traumatic stress disorder. Med Hypotheses 78(5):571–579, 2012 22365651

Waelde LC, Thompson L, Gallagher-Thompson D: A pilot study of a yoga and meditation intervention for dementia caregiver stress. J Clin Psychol 60(6):677–687, 2004 15141399

Wolff JL, Spillman BC, Freedman VA, et al: A national profile of family and unpaid caregivers who assist older adults with health care activities. JAMA Intern Med 176(3):372–379, 2016 26882031

PART III

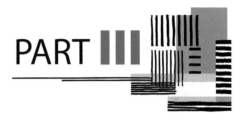

Education and Coaching

Section Editor:
Behdad Bozorgnia, M.D., M.A.P.P.

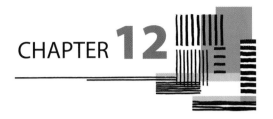

CHAPTER 12

Stress Management and Resiliency Training in Medical Internship

Aviva Teitelbaum, M.D.

Deanna C. Chaukos, M.D., F.R.C.P.C.

Editors' Introduction

This thoughtful and self-reflective chapter describes the problem of burnout among medical interns and describes one talented young physician who feels demoralized, insecure, and exhausted. She participates in and benefits substantially from the Stress Management and Resiliency Training for Residents (SMART-R) program, a very efficient and effective time-limited intervention for house officers. The typical reactions of some house officers to participating in this type of program and the rationale for the program are clearly explained and discussed.

SUMMARY

Lisa is a 26-year-old newly minted physician, currently in her first year of an internal medicine residency program in New York City. During the eighth month of her intern year, she finds herself physically and emotionally depleted, feeling that she cannot possibly give anything more to her patients and their families. She used to believe that becoming a physician was a noble calling. Now she doubts that she made the right career choice.

The Stress Management and Resiliency Training for Residents (SMART-R) program was implemented in Lisa's residency program, with the hopes of addressing burnout and bolstering resilience in first-year residents, a population at significant risk of burnout. The three tenets of the curriculum—elicitation of the relaxation response, stress awareness techniques, and adaptive strategies such as positive perspective taking—are incorporated into each of the three 2-hour sessions.

Person

Presentation

I feel like I'm in a long, dark tunnel, and there's no light at either end of it. It is February of my intern year, and I am so tired. I can't remember what my life was like before residency, nor can I imagine this year coming to an end. For the past 6 weeks, I've been working 80 hours a week on the inpatient medicine floors. Several of my patients have died, many have gotten better, and most have remained persistently ill. I'm ashamed to admit this, but I feel numb to it all; whether my patients die or are discharged, each demands a similar mountain of paperwork and collateral phone calls. I've been overlooking the distress and fear of my patients and their families and have been regarding them as obstacles to my getting home at the end of the day. How did I become so jaded?

Shortly after becoming an intern, one develops a reputation as a "black cloud" or "white cloud." The "white cloud" interns get few admissions on call and coast through their days, somehow spared of all the ways things could go wrong. I am not that kind of intern. I must have a massive thundercloud hanging over me: I get the most admissions while on call, I get assigned patients with the most difficult families, and my patients always seem to be the most medically unstable.

The best part of my day is leaving the hospital and going home to my quiet apartment. I cherish those few hours before bed each night. Whether I see a friend or zone out in front of the TV, I can try—for a few short hours—to forget that I have to return to the hospital at the crack of dawn the next day. For a few hours, I can pretend that I didn't spend my day around dying people. I try not to think about the impatient nurse who refused to get a set of vitals on my patient in respiratory distress. I can try to forget about being ripped apart by my attending for forgetting the treatment protocol for hospital-acquired pneumonia.

But in practice, I can't forget any of it. Despite feeling numb during the day, I take my work home with me: I ruminate about having put in the wrong medication or lab order, I worry I forgot to relay some critical piece of information to the incoming team, or perhaps I overemphasized the importance of something to the covering doctors that might cause them to miss something even more important. There is always so much that could go wrong, a calamity lurking around every corner. I don't think I used to feel this way.

When I was about age 8, I announced to my family that I wanted to become a cardiologist. I had a vague idea of what this meant—something to do with fixing hearts—but most importantly that's what my grandfather did, so I would do the same. Despite getting older and understanding what I'd have to sacrifice to pursue this noble career, I never deviated from my plan. In fact, I had romantic—and frankly grandiose—notions of my future: I imagined myself single-handedly saving the lives of my patients, all the while developing close relationships with them and their families, such that I'd become a dinner table name for many of them. I now look back and laugh at how far my fantasies were from the reality of my days as an intern physician. I now spend more time with a Hewlett Packard computer than with patients; my interactions with patients are generally thankless; and I am oftentimes unsuccessful in my attempts to help them.

I said good-bye to my grandfather during my third month of internship. He had a devastating stroke and died of a brain bleed. I remember getting the call from my mother as I was on night float. Despite how close I was to him, I didn't go to his funeral. I don't know if I could have gone, but at the time I thought I understood the culture of my residency program: work first, then personal matters. I remember finishing night float 2 weeks later, only to learn that my co-intern's grandparent had passed away. Ironically, I was the one to cover for her as she attended the funeral.

A few weeks ago, our program director announced that a resiliency curriculum was being added to our didactic schedule, and that it was mandatory to attend this 2-hour program every week for 3 weeks. In the e-mail, there was something about this program's goal of addressing physician burnout. I think I scoffed when I read the e-mail. How is a 6-hour course going to get rid of this feeling I'm carrying around with me? On top of that, 6 hours over the course of 3 weeks is valuable work time, and I know this will result in my leaving work later at the end of the day.

History/Background

Lisa has no prior psychiatric history: She has never been depressed or experienced episodes of psychosis or mania. She has never had a substance use disorder or a history of trauma. She has no family history of psychiatric illness. Her resilience has remained a defining and stable trait throughout her life; she manages high-stress situations and adverse conditions with thoughtfulness and poise. Lisa's negative self-concept, as evidenced by her narrative in the prior section, greatly contrasts with the way in which she presents herself in and outside work. She was beloved by her classmates in medical school for her sincerity and humor. Since beginning residency, she has developed solid relationships with her colleagues, who see her as an intelligent, hardworking team player.

FORMULATION

Not unlike many intern physicians, Lisa is suffering from burnout, which is considered a syndrome of dysfunction in three domains: emotional exhaustion, depersonalization, and reduced sense of personal accomplishment (Maslach 2003). Because of the demands of internship, she has started to feel emotionally depleted, numb to the distress of her patients and their families, and like a failure on all fronts. Burnout can manifest to different degrees, including as a manageable level of stress or even comorbid with a formal mood disorder. Although Lisa's feelings of physical and emotional depletion do not meet diagnostic criteria for a major depressive disorder or another mood disorder, her state of burnout is preventing her from practicing medicine to the best of her abilities and from feeling fulfilled in her career. Her own resilience has aided her in staying afloat during these trying times; however, resiliency is not a stable personality trait, and with enough stress and adversity, one can become less resilient and even more prone to negative manifestations of chronic stress.

INTERVENTION

SMART-R is a joint initiative that grew out of a collaboration between the Benson-Henry Institute for Mind Body Medicine (BHI) at Massachusetts General Hospital, a research and clinical institute for mind-body and resiliency training, and a group of interested residents in the departments of medicine and psychiatry. BHI, founded approximately 40 years ago, has developed an evidence-based resiliency training program called Stress Management and Resiliency Training: A Relaxation Response Resiliency Program (SMART-3RP). Over the past two decades, SMART-3RP has been studied and shown to have positive impacts on people with various chronic illnesses, including hypertension, chronic pain, and diabetes (Dusek et al. 2008; Samuelson et al. 2010). SMART-3RP has been implemented with diverse healthy populations as well, including in a Boston public school and the U.S. Armed Forces (Foret et al. 2012). The program has been shown to help individuals adapt to life's challenges, find meaning, and stay resilient. In 2012, the program was adapted for palliative care physicians and was shown to reduce reported stress (Mehta et al. 2016; Perez et al. 2015). Additionally, participants reported increased ability to find meaning in and take a positive perspective on their work.

SMART-3RP incorporates a three-pronged approach to resilience: 1) elicitation of the relaxation response, a physiological state conceptually opposite to the stress response, through the use of mind-body practices such as yoga and meditation (e.g., mantra, mindfulness, guided imagery); 2) development of stress awareness techniques and cognitive strategies for coping; and 3) development of adaptive perspectives. The program teaches numerous skills that independently have been shown to promote happiness and optimism (from positive psychology), to decrease depression (through cognitive-behavioral therapy techniques), and to improve life satisfaction (through a meditation practice). The SMART-R curriculum is an abbreviated version of SMART-3RP (Park et al. 2013), and the exercises have been adapted for the resident physician population.

The SMART-R curriculum is a preventive strategy to help trainees maintain and bolster resilience. It is important to note that this program is not a treatment for depression or other mental illness, and will not adequately serve as a replacement for secondary or tertiary care for depression or severe burnout. Physician well-being needs to be addressed at multiple levels, including that of adequate provision of mental health care for medical trainees (Daskivich et al. 2015).

Burnout describes a workplace phenomenon characterized by depersonalization, emotional exhaustion, and decreased sense of personal accomplishment (Maslach et al. 2001). Research has shown that burnout is highly prevalent among physicians (Dyrbye et al. 2014). Despite matriculating with higher resilience, medical trainees more commonly experience burnout than do their nonmedical peers (Dyrbye et al. 2014; Shanafelt et al. 2012), which suggests that the medical training and practice environment puts medical trainees at risk for burnout. The issue of burnout is significant, not only because of the risks to trainee well-being and trainees' future careers (Shanafelt et al. 2015), but also because of negative effects on the health care system and patient care (Beach et al. 2013; West et al. 2006). Burnout is not the only issue; perceived stress has been linked with depression and suicidal ideation in medical trainees (Shapiro et al. 2000). Physicians, perhaps more than most individuals, can appreciate that well-being is not simply the absence of pathology (Eckleberry-Hunt et al. 2009). SMART-R was therefore created to introduce resident physicians to adaptive coping strategies shown to bolster resilience, and to give residents permission to attend to their own well-being.

Why SMART-R Is a Positive Intervention

The SMART-R curriculum is divided into three sessions, each lasting 2 hours. Each session embeds exercises from each of the three pillars of the SMART-3RP: elicitation of the relaxation response, stress awareness techniques, and adaptive strategies.

CURRICULUM COMPONENTS

Practicing relaxation response techniques.   Each session includes different techniques to elicit the relaxation response, all of which involve creating and keeping a mental focus with an open and nonjudgmental attitude (e.g., guided imagery, body scan, single-pointed focus meditations).

Stress awareness techniques.   Through various behavioral strategies, participants are taught to examine the different ways in which stress has an impact on them, as well as to examine their personal responses to stress. During the program, these strategies are used to examine how stress affects one's thoughts, emotions, body, behavior, and relationships. The goal is for participants to recognize what core beliefs keep them in the stress response and make it more difficult for them to cope with stress.

Adaptive strategies.   With a new foundation of stress awareness, participants examine and practice adaptive strategies for stressful situations. These strategies are grouped into four categories: reappraisal and coping, positive perspectives, social connectedness, and healthy lifestyle behaviors.

Reappraisal and coping. The reappraisal approach is based in cognitive therapy, which recognizes the link between thoughts and emotions. Through a series of exercises, participants become more aware of their immediate responses to a stressor, as well as their corresponding negative thoughts, emotions, physical sensations, and behaviors. Participants learn how to reframe responses toward positive and adaptive thoughts, emotions, physical sensations, and behaviors. Through these exercises, participants will learn how to decrease the frequency of negative responses and to better cope with potential stressors.

Positive perspectives. These exercises draw on the field of positive psychology (Bolier et al. 2013; Duckworth et al. 2005), which emphasizes the expression of positive emotions and character strengths. Through a series of exercises and discussions, participants are challenged to find positive meaning, even in the midst of difficult situations, and to see stressors from an adaptive perspective.

Social connectedness. Activation of the stress response can fuel a sense of social isolation and disconnectedness, which in turn can propagate negative emotions. In this course, participants are encouraged to explore three main aspects of social connectedness: social support, empathy (for oneself and others), and helping others. Through various exercises, participants explore the different types of social support. They also practice effective listening skills, and explore how to elicit empathic thoughts, feelings, and behaviors.

Healthy lifestyle behaviors. In discussing healthy lifestyle behaviors, participants are encouraged to set goals of physical activity, nutrition and mindful eating, and sleep hygiene.

SESSIONS

Exercises from each of the three prongs of the program are integrated into each 2-hour session. The sessions typically occur weekly over 3 weeks, although some residency programs have spread them over a longer period due to scheduling challenges.

Session 1.   The goals of session 1 are for participants to learn how to elicit the relaxation response, to start to look at how stress impacts the individual, and to explore individual stressors and the resources available to cope with stress. The session starts with an overview of the evidence base for mindfulness training for doctors (Krasner et al. 2009) and the concept of resiliency. In this session, participants are introduced to the concept of the relaxation response by learning a few basic guided meditations. Participants are guided to develop awareness of stress-linked thoughts, emotions, behaviors, and physical experiences. The concept of social support is introduced through a discussion of the different types of social support (emotional, informational, tangible, affirmational, and belonging-type supports). Finally, participants learn an approach to goal setting that facilitates taking inventory of priorities in life, and aligning these to goals set in residency training.

Session 2.   In session 2, participants examine how stress affects both the mind and the body, a concept that physicians often discuss with their patients but may neglect for themselves. Participants begin with a guided body scan meditation. This practice of "noticing," or observation, is one that physicians cultivate as a clinical skill in medicine, used on a daily basis when making phenomenological observations of their patients. By turning this skill inward, participants are encouraged to nurture and care for themselves, thus becoming more attuned and connected physicians. Participants discuss ways in which the relaxation response practice can extend throughout the day, not simply during meditation. Then, participants are introduced to the concepts of negative automatic thoughts and thought distortions, and consider how these apply to common experiences in residency. Once participants identify common thought distortions embedded in their own thoughts, beliefs, and behaviors, they are encouraged to identify new ways of coping with challenging situations, by practicing positive perspective–taking strategies. The discussion of adaptive perspectives is expanded by examining the impact of optimistic and pessimistic perspectives; learning how these can influence resiliency and stress, respectively; and considering methods of understanding the underlying fears that drive pessimistic thinking.

Session 3.   In session 3, participants are introduced to guided imagery, which utilizes the power of visualization and imagination to evoke a sense of well-being and encourage insight. Participants explore meaning-finding in their work, and more broadly in their lives. The role of empathy for self and others in building and maintaining resiliency is emphasized. Participants share their individual ways for finding meaning, such as through creative expression, the arts, athletics, and comedy. The role of humor in medicine is explored—including conflicting feelings about dark humor, process and comic release, and the importance of knowing oneself. The importance of ongoing reflection is emphasized in order to create meaning from daily events that would otherwise have gone unnoticed. This third session ends with reexamination of participants' initial goals, reflection on lessons learned, and considering how participants can emit their "idealized self."

Implementation Process

SMART-R is implemented for resident physicians with very busy schedules, and there are important challenges to implementation. Time is an important challenge. In order to accommodate residents' schedules, the program length was abbreviated from the original 16-hour SMART-3RP course. The shortened 6-hour SMART-R program thereby serves as a "tasting menu" of positive strategies. Residents must feel freed from their usual responsibilities to attend these sessions, and the curriculum should not feel like an additional burden or task. This can be achieved by ensuring that resident time is protected, embedding the curriculum into the preexisting resident didactic schedule, and replacing some other expectations.

The second implementation challenge involves ensuring that the group facilitator is someone uninvolved in resident evaluation. A facilitator can be an individual with group therapy experience, a personal meditation practice, or interest in group dynamics, or simply be someone who is curious, flexible, and engaged with trainees. These groups require a facilitator who can set the tone for self-reflection and nonjudgment. The group environment also needs to respect resident privacy; as such, group facilitators should not be faculty who directly evaluate residents.

Finally, an important consideration for implementation is the culture of the residency program adopting the curriculum. Like all interventions that aim to change an established culture, programs that address physician well-being can come up against resistance, which is in part influenced by the "hidden curriculum" in medicine—an ingrained culture of stoicism, prioritization of work above all else (including one's own health), and perseverance as a sign of strength. Thus, before a wellness curriculum can be adopted in a residency program, it is important to understand the culture from within the program.

In smaller residency programs, it can be difficult to identify faculty who are uninvolved in evaluating residents to run SMART-R groups; thus, it can be helpful to identify faculty champions willing to work with residents in different specialty programs. This strategy also allows for specialties to collaborate together in a resilience curriculum aimed at fostering trainee well-being. To date, SMART-R has been implemented for internal medicine, psychiatry, neurology, and pediatrics residents in urban and rural programs of diverse sizes (Chaukos et al. 2017, 2018).

OUTCOME

Although I was skeptical, I attended the SMART-R course. During the first session, I was vocal about how frustrated I felt to be told I had to attend a mandatory wellness program, which seems oxymoronic. The group facilitator began by discussing the importance of intentionally pausing during our day, and taking a moment to be with our breath, as a way to shift our focus.

"I don't mean to be rude, but it feels counterproductive to slow down when my work keeps piling up. A pause is one thing, but these 2 hours are a lot of time to take away from my workday. It may not seem like much to you, but it means I leave here behind on my work, and I'm stuck at work until late."

"Thanks for your thoughts," said the group facilitator. "Do these sentiments resonate with anyone else?"

Everyone nodded.

Despite my protests, I completed the 6-hour SMART-R course and discovered that it did not in fact waste my time. Much to my surprise, I looked forward to this 2-hour pause every week. I discovered that I am not as alone as I thought: my co-interns also experience burnout, and they also regard themselves as black clouds. I learned that I am not defined by my negative thoughts or experiences, or by the stress of intern year. I had felt ashamed of my thoughts, such that having them meant that I was not a good doctor. It was a relief to share how alone I feel, and to learn that the group of people I spend most of my time with feel the same way. In addition to recognizing the universality of our experience, we spent some time learning about mindfulness strategies that are helpful to use when working on a busy medicine floor. We talked about the importance of humor in medicine, and of our connection to one another. We also looked at negative automatic thoughts that are specific to the internship experience, and started to challenge those thoughts. I started realizing that the way I see myself is not consistent with the way others see me: my co-interns were shocked to learn that I think of myself as incompetent, and collectively told me that their impression was that I am exactly the opposite. Even though intern year remains difficult, and this course did not change that fact, I began to deliberately take notice of small acts of kindness, as well as the things and people I feel grateful for. For example, yesterday I helped a patient express to his family what was important to him at the end of his life. Afterward, he took my hand, and said thank you. This experience made me feel connected, and reconnected me to my values of humanity in medicine.

Symptoms and Positive Experiences, Strengths, and Satisfaction

One of the most cathartic aspects of the SMART-R program was recognizing that I am not alone. I felt a great deal of shame about the type of physician I had become, and about how far that was from the life-saving, kindhearted, involved, nurturing physician I thought I was going to be—the kind of physician my childhood self imagined my grandpa to be. Once I started to talk about how I was feeling toward my patients, how overwrought I felt, and how disappointed I was in myself, most of the group members related to my experience. And with that, the shame began to dissipate.

The SMART-R program encouraged me to try to shift my perspective. Many of us were accustomed to focusing on the negative aspects of situations, or the areas in which we had little control, rather than reflecting on what was positive about the situation and where there was room to make a change. During the program, we talked about feeling powerless as interns, having little autonomy, always having to answer to some superior. The group facilitator pointed out that while that was true, we were forgetting about the medical student experience: that as residents we have the power to model positive behavior and make an important impact on medical education. With this exercise, we were encouraged to make positive changes in the academic experience of the medical student—something that we had the ability to impact.

The introduction to positive psychology strategies helped me recognize that positive psychology is not about ignoring negative emotion; rather, by integrating mind-body strategies, I became more aware of both positive and negative emotions, and the ways they were inadvertently impacting my perceptions and behavior. I learned that time for mourning and reflection on loss is integral, and that rumination and worry are different from mindful reflection. Rumination was further isolating me, whereas mindful reflection helped me reach out to my co-residents and connect to community in the face of loss.

Assessment of the Patient's Progress and Response

As a result of attending the SMART-R program, Lisa made some changes in her life. She began to incorporate short mindfulness practices into her daily routine. She tried to eat one item of food in a mindful manner each day, paying attention to the full experience of eating her food, rather than rushing through it as she typically did. Prior to entering her patients' rooms, Lisa would do a short breathing exercise as she was washing her hands. She discovered that these few seconds of mindful breathing put her in a frame of mind in which she was alert, attentive, and aware of the full experience of being with the patient. She started to keep an appreciation journal: on her subway ride home, she would list three things for which she was grateful that day. With each entry, she felt increasingly grateful, and she wanted to share her gratitude with others. She became more involved in teaching medical students and more open to engaging with other hospital staff, rather than rushing by, fueled by her mission to get out of the hospital as soon as possible. With these small changes, Lisa began to feel more at home in her place of work.

Why the Positive Intervention Mattered

Residency is a time of great personal challenge and change, when young professionals develop habits that can become long-standing practices. Thus, it is an important time to implement positive strategies that maintain well-being. For physicians, well-being is influenced greatly by the ability to connect with purpose. In this case example, the positive intervention allowed Lisa to pause and reflect on how stress had influenced her emotions, thoughts, and behaviors, and helped guide her toward a deliberate practice that better serves her and her patients.

TAKE-HOME POINTS

- Deliberate practice is part of professionalism in medicine. Physicians and other clinicians have a duty to themselves and their patients to have a means for self-reflection and self-care.

- The practice of medicine is wrought with existential and philosophical quandaries. Positive psychology practices can help by fostering connection, meaning, and realistic optimism.

- It is important to recognize that burnout is a complex work environment problem that requires a systematic approach. Although individual practices alone are not enough to tackle this complex problem, they can help individual physicians cope with the dehumanizing and exhausting aspects of the work.

- Positive psychology practices implemented by physicians can help improve well-being for both physicians and their patients.

REFERENCES

Beach MC, Roter D, Korthuis PT, et al: A multicenter study of physician mindfulness and health care quality. Ann Fam Med 11(5):421–428, 2013 24019273

Bolier L, Haverman M, Westerhof GJ, et al: Positive psychology interventions: a meta-analysis of randomized controlled studies. BMC Public Health 13(1):119, 2013 23390882

Chaukos D, Cromartie D, et al: Stress management and resiliency training program for residents implementation toolkit. Adopted as a peer-reviewed model curriculum by the American Association of Psychiatry Residency Training Directors Curriculum Committee, March 7, 2017. Available at: www.AADPRT.org.

Chaukos D, Chad-Friedman E, Mehta DH, et al: SMART-R: a prospective cohort study of a resilience curriculum for residents by residents. Acad Psychiatry 42:78–83, 2018

Daskivich TJ, Jardine DA, Tseng J, et al: Promotion of wellness and mental health awareness among physicians in training: perspective of a national, multispecialty panel of residents and fellows. J Grad Med Educ 7(1):143–147, 2015 26217450

Duckworth AL, Steen TA, Seligman MEP: Positive psychology in clinical practice. Annu Rev Clin Psychol 1:629–651, 2005 17716102

Dusek JA, Hibberd PL, Buczynski B, et al: Stress management versus lifestyle modification on systolic hypertension and medication elimination: a randomized trial. J Altern Complement Med 14(2):129–138, 2008 18315510

Dyrbye LN, West CP, Satele D, et al: Burnout among U.S. medical students, residents, and early career physicians relative to the general U.S. population. Acad Med 89(3):443–451, 2014 24448053

Eckleberry-Hunt J, Van Dyke A, Lick D, et al: Changing the conversation from burnout to wellness: physician well-being in residency training programs. J Grad Med Educ 1(2):225–230, 2009 21975983

Foret MM, Scult M, Wilcher M, et al: Integrating a relaxation response-based curriculum into a public high school in Massachusetts. J Adolesc 35(2):325–332, 2012 21893336

Krasner MS, Epstein RM, Beckman H, et al: Association of an educational program in mindful communication with burnout, empathy, and attitudes among primary care physicians. JAMA 302(12):1284–1293, 2009 19773563

Maslach C: Burnout: The Cost of Caring. Cambridge, MA, Malor Books, 2003

Maslach C, Schaufeli WB, Leiter MP: Job burnout. Annu Rev Psychol 52:397–422, 2001 11148311

Mehta DH, Perez GK, Traeger L, et al: Building resiliency in a palliative care team: a pilot study. J Pain Symptom Manage 51(3):604–608, 2016 26550936

Park ER, Traeger L, Vranceanu A-M, et al: The development of a patient-centered program based on the relaxation response: the Relaxation Response Resiliency Program (3RP). Psychosomatics 54(2):165–174, 2013 23352048

Perez GK, Haime V, Jackson V, et al: Promoting resiliency among palliative care clinicians: stressors, coping strategies, and training needs. J Palliat Med 18(4):332–337, 2015 25715108

Samuelson M, Foret M, Baim M, et al: Exploring the effectiveness of a comprehensive mind-body intervention for medical symptom relief. J Altern Complement Med 16(2):187–192, 2010 20180692

Shanafelt TD, Boone S, Tan L, et al: Burnout and satisfaction with work-life balance among U.S. physicians relative to the general U.S. population. Arch Intern Med 172(18):1377–1385, 2012 22911330

Shanafelt TD, Hasan O, Dyrbye LN, et al: Changes in burnout and satisfaction with work-life balance in physicians and the general U.S. working population between 2011 and 2014. Mayo Clin Proc 90(12):1600–1613, 2015 26653297

Shapiro SL, Shapiro DE, Schwartz GE: Stress management in medical education: a review of the literature. Acad Med 75(7):748–759, 2000 10926029

West CP, Huschka MM, Novotny PJ, et al: Association of perceived medical errors with resident distress and empathy: a prospective longitudinal study. JAMA 296(9):1071–1078, 2006 16954486

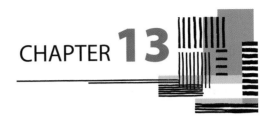

CHAPTER 13

Acting "As If" in Executive Coaching

Shannon M. Polly, M.A.P.P., PCC

Kathryn H. Britton, M.A.P.P.

Editors' Introduction

This rich and nuanced account of a coaching intervention de-scribes the conceptual background for coaching, distinguishing it from treatment, and provides a thorough description of this technique. Three cases—an individual and two group-oriented examples—provide interesting details about how people used the intervention to help develop specific behaviors they set as goals in work and other settings. The specificity of the goals and of the intervention allows the coach to employ a variety of very effective techniques that resonate with the reader and remind us how we all have areas in which we would like to grow.

Coaches, like clinicians, work with people who want to become better versions of themselves. Coaches do not deal with diagnosed psychiatric problems, but their clients often come with beliefs that they want to reframe or with goals that they are not sure how to achieve. Coaches use many of the same tools that clinicians use: listening closely, reflecting back what they hear, brain-storming best next steps, and suggesting ways to interpret events in more constructive lights.

Coaches who draw on positive psychology often emphasize the following in their work:

- *Strengths.* It is typically more productive to enhance strengths and employ them more broadly than it is to focus on weaknesses. In our work, we focus primarily on character strengths (Niemiec 2014; Peterson and Seligman 2004; Polly and Britton 2015).
- *Growth mindsets.* Skills, behaviors, knowledge, and even intelligence are not fixed. They can be enhanced through effort, perseverance, and dealing with obstacles (Dweck 2007).
- *Self-efficacy.* There are ways to intentionally enhance people's beliefs so individuals are able to positively affect circumstances in their lives (Bandura 1977).

Coaching has also benefited from many positive psychology approaches that originated in clinical psychology, including the following:

- *Narrative psychology.* It benefits clients to tell stories about their lives, generating insights, coherence, and recognition of the potential for positivity (Tarragona 2013).
- *Solution focus.* Shifting clients' focus from problems to solutions helps them recognize strengths that already exist and imagine paths to solutions that work (Berg and Szabo 2005; de Shazer and Dolan 2007; Iveson et al. 2012; Terni 2015).

A wide range of coaching tools and practices are based on these beliefs. Some of these are described in books (Biswas-Diener 2010; Biswas-Diener and Dean 2007; Oren et al. 2007). Wharton Executive Education has collected more than 80 activities that they call Nano Tools for Leaders (Wharton Executive Education 2017). With difficulty, we selected one practice—acting "as if"—to discuss in this chapter because this practice helps people try on new ways of acting. This approach can easily be tailored to match the needs of very different clients, including those in clinical settings.

In this chapter, we discuss the background of acting "as if" as a coaching strategy, explore its active ingredients, and illustrate it in action with three cases. We chose to present multiple clients to illustrate ways to tailor the practice to meet different needs.

BACKGROUND: ACTING "AS IF"

Acting "as if" is a behavioral intervention that helps people try on different ways of behaving and, by doing so, update their mental pictures of themselves.

Although this approach can be traced back to acting teachers, especially Konstantin Stanislavsky (Stanislavski 1936/1989a, 1936/1989b), many psychologists have recognized the benefits of exploring new roles to aid development, including Alfred Adler (1938, 1964; Watts et al. 2005), Daryl Bem (1972), Albert Bandura (1977), Mark Carich (1997), and Carol Dweck (2007).

One of the authors of this chapter (SMP) learned the actor's toolkit by studying Stanislavsky in college and drama school. The techniques she learned as an actor are just as useful to ordinary people off stage. With imagination and coaching, people can act "as if" they already were the way they want to be.

According to Harold Mosak's explanation of Adlerian psychotherapy, as repeated by Carlson and Sperry (1998), "When someone has difficulty acting prosocially, that is, speaking assertively or responding with some measure of empathy, the clinician might encourage them to act 'as if' they were assertive or empathic several times a day until the next session. The rationale for this reconstruction strategy is that as someone begins to act differently and to feel differently, they become a different person" (p. 73).

Social psychologist Bem (1972) stated that humans form conclusions about themselves by observing themselves in the same way they form conclusions by observing others. Acting "as if" gives people opportunities to enact best possible outcomes or to create new stories about their lives. Asking people to pretend can help them get past resistance to change because it is temporary and merely an experiment. As they observe themselves behaving in new ways, they update their mental models about what they can do.

Coaching mentors have told us not to use the term *role-play* because clients may viscerally object to the idea of performing. However, when we ask a client to "try on" a conversation with the boss about reducing hours, words flow. The future conversation appears less daunting.

In human development, people venture from who they are right now into who they are not yet but could be. Russian psychologist Lev Vygotsky (1978) calls that new territory the "zone of proximal development." The acquisition of new knowledge is dependent on previous learning as well as "trying on" new behaviors, often reflected back to us by the people around us. If a baby says "ba-ba," we don't say, "Nope, that's not it. Try again!" We say, "Bottle! Look, honey, she just said 'bottle'!" As adults, we help children grow into what they can become. Similarly, coaches and clinicians can encourage clients to "try on" new ways of behaving, then help them see new images of themselves. Venturing into their own zones of proximal development, clients expand their ideas about who they are and what is possible. Cathy Salit (2016) describes applications of the zone of proximal development concept to augment workplace performance.

Table 13–1 summarizes some contributions that acting "as if" can make to client well-being. The coach may or may not want to describe these qualities to a client, depending on the individual's curiosity about why acting "as if" is so beneficial. It can be helpful to have clients take the Values in Action (VIA) Survey of Character Strengths (VIA Institute on Character 2017) prior to beginning this intervention so they will be ready to use the language of strengths when talking about desired outcomes and behaviors to practice.

Intervention

Clinical practitioners familiar with psychodrama or play therapy will recognize the overlap between the acting "as if" technique and the work they do. Although many sample sizes are small, the literature shows strong results for using psychodrama and its positive impact on psychological well-being, specifically on autonomy, positive relations, self-acceptance, environmental mastery, purposeful growth, and meaningful living (Nikzadeh and Soudani 2016). Acting "as if" differs from psychodrama in that it can be leveraged in a clinical or coaching setting and is often implemented at the client's work or home. The intervention can be tailored to the client, and it should follow this basic structure:

- Determining objectives by identifying the qualities the client wishes to enhance
- Using scaling questions in order to set a baseline and track progress
- Identifying at least one paragon of each desired quality
- Leveraging imagination to act "as if" the client has already enhanced the desired qualities
- Reflecting on the experience of acting "as if" and how changed behaviors have impacted the client and other people

Determining Objectives

Through open-ended questions, the coach helps the client explore the desired characteristics or end state the client wishes to achieve. Clients often want to enhance performance in a certain way in specific situations. Examples of questions that might be helpful appear in Table 13–2.

Actors create objectives that control the way they develop particular roles by thinking about what the character wants and needs. Thinking about the same questions, clients similarly articulate broad overall objectives, such as "I want to be an effective leader," and then translate them into objectives for particular situations, such as "I want to be heard and respected in the meeting with my peers on Friday."

TABLE 13–1. Positive qualities built by acting "as if"

Positive quality	Description	Source	How acting "as if" helps
Self-efficacy	The personal belief that one can succeed in a particular situation.	Bandura 1977	Gives people a safe way to venture beyond areas of certainty, and to stretch abilities. Leads to personal mastery experiences.
Growth mindset	The personal belief that learning is more important than looking smart/good. Associated with greater ability to take risks and learn by doing.	Dweck 2007	Helps people try on growth mindsets in a safe space. Once they see benefits of a growth mindset in one domain, they often can extend it to others. Coaches can help them interpret difficulties as welcome opportunities to learn new approaches.
Character strengths	Human qualities valued across time, nationalities, religions.	Peterson and Seligman 2004	Bolsters signature strengths and builds lesser strengths.

TABLE 13–2. Coaching questions used with the acting "as if" intervention

Step	Possible coaching questions
Determining objectives	How would you behave if your life were unfolding exactly as it should?
	What quality or qualities would show that you've made progress toward your deepest goals?
	If you exhibited this quality on a daily basis, what would it look like?
	When have you exhibited this quality in the past?
	What would this quality look like in your life?
	How would other people notice that you had this quality?
Using scaling questions	Where are you right now with this quality? Please give me a number from 1 to 10, where 1 means "hardly at all" and 10 means "fully there."
	(Initially) Great! What puts you at a 4 and not a 3 or a 2?
	(Later) What helped you move from 4 to 6?
	(Later) What differences do you think people around you have observed?
Identifying paragons	When have you yourself exhibited this quality?
	Who do you know who has this quality? Consider family, colleagues, teachers.
	Who do you know from history or popular culture who has this quality?
Leveraging imagination	What does it look like to have this quality?
	What does it feel like in your body to have this quality?
	What other qualities that you have already could support this quality?
Reflecting on progress	When are you exhibiting the new behavior?
	What opportunities have you missed?
	What changes have the people around you observed?

Using Scaling Questions

Scaling questions, also shown in Table 13–2, come from solution-focused therapy and coaching (de Shazer and Dolan 2007; Iveson et al. 2012; Terni 2015). They help clients capture a baseline sense of strengths that already exist.

Scaling questions build self-efficacy by turning the client's attention toward strengths already possessed and past successes. The coach can remember the scaling number and bring it up later after asking the scaling question again to help clients see progress.

Identifying Paragons

Acting "as if" can be enhanced by recalling examples of the desired behavior in action. What does it look like to be brave, thoughtful, strategic, influential, or whatever qualities the client decided to build?

It can be helpful for the coach to first ask clients to recollect times when they have been their own paragons. One client described herself as a mother bear when it came to advocating for treatment of her son's health problems, but she had difficulty speaking up in meetings. When she acted "as if" she were the mother bear in her next meeting, she found her voice was stronger and she could exhibit the once elusive ability to assert herself at work.

It can also be powerful to ask clients for paragons in their families or among people they know well, such as colleagues and teachers. Finally, they may look to admired figures from history or the popular culture. It is helpful for them to identify multiple paragons to emulate in different situations. For famous paragons, it may be possible to find speeches or quotations that clients can read aloud to try out acting like them. Table 13–2 lists some questions for helping clients identify paragons.

Leveraging Imagination

To many people, the expression "Fake it 'til you make it" implies inauthenticity. However, most people as children played by pretending to be someone they were not (yet). The coach can help people feel safe enough to play with extensions to their current identities. Some clients need only a reminder of what it was like to play as a child and how playing is inherently natural and fun. Others need to hear about research on the benefits of play for children and for adults. Pretend play has been shown to improve creativity, language and literacy, and executive function. There are social and emotional benefits as well. Pretend play helps with navigating interpersonal interactions, socialization, social understanding and coping, and emotion regulation (Brown and Vaughan 2009). Research by Nikzadeh and Soudani (2016) shows that role-play, specifically, teaches empathy and understanding of different perspectives. It improves interpersonal and communication skills.

Lev Vygotsky (1978) wrote, "In play it is as though [the child] were a head taller than himself. As in the focus of a magnifying glass, play contains all developmental tendencies in a condensed form and is itself a major source of development" (p. 102). Humans do not grow too old to benefit from play.

Clients can leverage their character strengths through play. People who are aware of their own top character strengths can play with ways to use them in new contexts and in new ways. What would it mean to use kindness and fairness to become a better leader? What would it mean to use humility and perspective to give more compelling presentations? These are open-ended questions that can lead to experimental behaviors in the coaching context that might then lead to trying on changes in other contexts.

Notably, many clients go right to their bottom-ranked strengths with concern. Here's a dialogue that might occur between client and coach:

CLIENT: How can I develop this particular strength that is number 24 on my list?

COACH: Pretend that you have that strength already. Act "as if" you are kind [or forgiving, or curious, or…]. In your next meeting, try acting "as if" you have that strength.

CLIENT: But how do I do that if I don't know how?

COACH: Make it up. You have probably observed someone acting that way in your life.

When it comes to acting "as if," some clients need a little help. One way to act "as if" is to read a piece of literature or a speech that embodies that strength. In self-efficacy terms, that means gaining some vicarious mastery by behaving just like someone who has already achieved mastery (Bandura 1977). We recommend that clients not merely read the pieces silently to themselves. Reading silently is just taking in the text with the eyes. Reading aloud sharpens focus, connects the reader to emotions, stimulates imagination, and involves the whole body.

Character Strengths Matter: How to Live a Full Life (Polly and Britton 2015) includes a speech for each of the 24 character strengths (Peterson and Seligman 2004). For example, a client working on gratitude might read aloud Lou Gehrig's good-bye speech, whereas one working on forgiveness might read aloud Portia's "quality of mercy" speech from *Merchant of Venice.*

As our clients imagine their way into particular roles, we frequently ask them to change the way they act physically. We might ask them, "How would you stand? How would you move? What would be the tenor of your voice? How would you make eye contact?"

One client read the Joan of Arc speech in *Character Strengths Matter* with a speaking voice and physical presence too small and quiet for the role. The coach asked her to go to the far side of a large room and think about how to physically embody Joan's signature strengths. Focusing on bravery and wisdom, the client stood up straighter, had a wider physical stance, and looked ahead rather than at the ground. When she tried the speech again, she was physically bigger but still vocally quiet. The coach then suggested that she imagine her audience was hard of hearing so she needed to speak at her top volume to be heard. She thought of the voice she used to call her children home. By channeling the character of Saint Joan and employing her own "mommy" voice, she went from being a timid speaker to being a commanding one.

Reflecting on Progress

After clients have been imagining, playing, reading aloud, and practicing, it can be helpful to explore how far they have come. The coach might ask scaling questions again.

Some clients also benefit from doing a self-evaluation in a daily journal. This gives them a chance to build their self-awareness. We also ask them to solicit feedback from colleagues or close family members. Possible reflection questions appear in Table 13–2.

CASE HISTORIES

The following case histories show applications of acting "as if" with three relatively successful people who were trying in different ways to expand their roles and enhance the way they appeared to others at work. The settings are different: the first involved individual one-on-one coaching, the second involved group coaching with a number of peers working on similar concerns, and the third involved a leadership program involving improvisation followed by group and individual coaching. The second and third cases demonstrate leveraging the collective support of others to build competence and self-efficacy.

The names and details have been changed to protect client confidentiality. Rather than describe problems faced by clients, we describe the goals they seek to attain, because coaches are not trained to identify problems that need therapy.

Individual Coaching: Eric

Eric is the general counsel at a law firm. He has a number of strengths that have contributed to his success there (and some of them he has overused): judgment, love of learning, kindness, humor, perspective, and prudence. His manager felt that Eric needed to increase his confidence to present to his board of directors with adequate gravitas. Eric accepted his manager's suggested leadership coaching because he knew that becoming a more accomplished speaker was important for his career trajectory, including an impending promotion opportunity. Thinking about being in front of the board made him somewhat anxious.

Eric met with a coach for 12 sessions. First came some preliminary exploration that established a baseline with questions like "When you have presented to the board in the past, what actual thoughts went through your head?" He mentioned that the board members were more experienced than he was, they were from very powerful companies, and he was younger than the other people in the room.

Because Eric was a practicing attorney, the coach leveraged that experience to ask him to act "as if" he were in court arguing a case for the opposite side, from the viewpoint "Why is Eric the most qualified person in the room to be talking?" Eric effectively argued that he knew the most about the subject because he had been working on it the longest. In fact, he knew even more about it than his boss. It was this initial trial of the acting "as if" technique linked to his previous experience that led the coach to believe that this was the best choice of intervention for Eric. In addition, because his goals were specifically related to presenting in front of the board of directors, this technique proved a direct link to the goals he wanted to achieve.

Other baseline questions included these: "What topics are you excited to present to the board?" "When do you think you are most successful in presentations?" "Where is your area for growth in making presentations?" It emerged that Eric was bored with presenting the material. If he was bored presenting, the audience would be bored listening. Therefore, Eric needed to make presenting the information interesting to himself so he could convey that interest to his audience. This took some exploration. He tried a few different versions of his presentation in different roles. Because it was shortly after the national holiday, Eric thought to take on Martin Luther King, Jr., as his first role. His initial attempt was a bit flat, so the coach asked him to try other roles, such as a Baptist preacher, to get increased vocal variety, and a man talking to a friend, to sound conversational rather than formal. What finally worked best for Eric was to act "as if" he were really excited about the topic. Sometimes focusing on a general characteristic works better than trying to be like someone else.

For additional practice, Eric read speeches from *Character Strengths Matter* (Polly and Britton 2015) for the character strengths he decided he wanted to build: bravery, social intelligence, and zest. From the gravitas of Martin Luther King, Jr., to the zest of the preacher, to the energy and vocal variety of a favorite schoolteacher, Eric found that he had many more "notes" to play in his presentation.

In the week leading up to the meeting, Eric practiced up to an hour per day by himself, an hour with his coach, and 3 hours the day before with his manager. Having some of these additional coaching tools added to the ways in which he was able to prepare the material. This much practice might make some clients wooden and over-rehearsed, which luckily did not happen with Eric. He also taped himself, working diligently to get a take that conveyed all the characteristics he wanted. He listened to the presentation recording be-cause he said, "I wanted to know it like you know your favorite song." Re-cording the presentation and listening to playbacks was Eric's own idea. We do not usually suggest it, because it makes some people more self-conscious.

Eric felt that the presentation for the board and other committees went well. His boss was pleased with the outcome. Eric has become more confi-dent speaking in interorganizational meetings. The coach observed greater physical confidence in his posture and voice and more psychological confi-dence in his abilities.

Going forward, Eric feels able to prepare for these presentations on his own without the help of a coach or his boss. When asked how this process affected him, he reflects,

> I feel more confident, and it is self-fulfilling....I feel like I can do that again when I prepare. I should be confident because I did great last time. It is the subconscious reinforcement that occurs....I can meet my goal in the future, of course I can....I met it last time.

Acting "as if" worked well for Eric. Even though the intervention in this situation was more directive than is usual with coaching, Eric was able to make the process his own by choosing which role worked best for him and devising his own process for rehearsing.

Group Coaching: Nathan

Nathan is a British manager in a credit card company. He is thoughtful and well spoken but generally chooses not to speak in large groups because of his stam-mer. He joined a coaching group with colleagues all concerned with building leadership skills. He leveraged his strengths of wisdom, fairness, and bravery in this intervention.

The coach asked each member of the group to perform a scene depicting a significant moment in his or her life, and then modeled this activity by en-acting a moment that showed more vulnerability than they were used to see-ing in typical work scenarios. Nathan decided to reveal his struggle with his stammer, which helped the whole group feel more comfortable sharing vul-nerabilities. When asked why he chose to do that, he replied,

I spoke then because I felt it was the right time to do so. I don't know why. It was a break-the-ice scenario. People didn't want to be vulnerable. In a work context, you are taught not to be vulnerable.... I had something I thought people could relate to. I showed vulnerability in the first discussion, and it wasn't shut down. I felt comfortable that I could trust the people there.

The coach asked the people in the group to play other roles outside their comfort zones: as a member of the other gender, as a brash executive, and as an exuberant teenager. Nathan shared an insight about the challenge that most clients face when they are asked to act "as if":

The role-playing was extremely uncomfortable. The first one…was like being fake.... You have got to become somebody else in that scenario. One of the key things I got from it is…you can show up as who you need to be, but still be yourself. And it makes no sense. But you can still have your strengths, your empathy.... Your personality can still come through regardless of who you need to be in that scenario.

Acting "as if" often requires people to act in ways that initially feel inauthentic. Coaches can help clients give themselves permission to do it anyway to see if the behavior can become authentic with practice. As Nathan pointed out, that often means connecting the new behavior to strengths and positive qualities that individuals already recognize as their own.

Solution-focused questions caused group members to recall times when they had expressed naturally occurring strengths in the past. Nathan mentioned that at home he had no problem acting bravely. If his kids were hurt or he disagreed with his wife, he had no problem standing up for himself.

Nathan was preparing for meetings in which he needed to let some employees go and reassure others about their ongoing roles in the company. He decided that the constellation of strengths he needed to leverage in these meetings included kindness and social intelligence. He practiced acting "as if" he had these strengths in combination. After the meetings, Nathan felt that he had been able to let some employees go with grace and kindness and to soothe the fears of the ones remaining with the company.

As we finished the coaching group, Nathan had a final presentation to make to the group. Despite reporting being terrified to get up in front of the group, he not only presented well and fielded questions, but he did not stammer once. When later asked how he did this, he replied,

A few times I thought I was going to block [*involuntary pause*] but I didn't....
When I came in that morning,…I felt horrible. I think you helped calm me down [when you said], "It's fine. And it can be normal." The group gave me the support that meant that I didn't have to be so nervous. I didn't have to think about stammering. I stammer less when someone knows I have a stammer.

They won't think it's me being rude; they will understand and take the time to listen.

Nathan decided that he was not going to share in every work situation the fact that he stammers, but he would consider being vulnerable in that and other ways if the situation called for it. He saw the benefit for a leader to share a struggle rather than pretend to have everything under control. He was surprised to become a leader in the group from making that choice. Asked at the end of the coaching to reflect in a journal or with a colleague on the biggest shift he made, Nathan described a mindset change:

> Now I'll start from "yes" or "why not?" rather than "why?" I have more of a positive outlook. I can help other people. I got to where I am because of me. And the work I do. And I shouldn't undervalue that. If I can help others, then I should.

The intervention was a successful one because Nathan came to understand that the technique did not mean that he was being inauthentic. He had a dramatic shift in mindset that enriched his performance and attitude at work. The tool was helpful even with a relatively intractable speech impediment.

Leadership Program With Improvisation: Vanessa

Vanessa is a senior manager at a high-tech company. Only a few years away from potential retirement, she felt that her supervisors (including her direct supervisor, Rich) were not putting her forward for promotion because of her age. Vanessa was feeling stuck. She did not see anything she could do about it.

Vanessa was nominated for a leadership development program that included three training sessions, group coaching sessions (6 hours), and individual coaching (6 hours). The training sessions used improvisational tools to explore the strength of bravery. Participants were challenged to act "as if" they were brave, flexible, creative, collaborative, and open-minded. Vanessa applied her strengths of zest, social intelligence, and humor/playfulness in this intervention. She then worked with a coach to figure out ways to apply what she learned in the improvisation sessions to her own situation.

Vanessa found other people whose performance she admired in the leadership program, people who could serve as her paragons. Here is how she described the program:

> It taught you how to reach out, build relationships, and recognize the strengths in other people you want to learn more about or emulate. A lot was looking at and seeing the positives that other people brought and [considering,] "How do I be like them?" I was looking at my peers and thinking, "How do they act in real time?" Their ability to observe, listen, and then articulate direction back—

I thought that was pretty amazing. I guess the first session I wanted to be like them....I still have a lot of growing to do, but I can be not just like them, but I can be my own version of them.

Vanessa used individual coaching sessions to address the obstacles that had kept her from seeking a promotion. She explained,

When you [the coach] asked, "Why aren't you going directly to Rich?" I don't know why I had that shield up before. I relied on the hierarchy here. I paid attention to that. You made me think about breaking down barriers. They were barriers I perceived were there. I built the wall. I got some not-so-great feedback that I thought was real: Rich didn't see [my promotion potential]. I was OK with that. The coaching gave me this strength...I guess I never thought about it before.

It is common for people in business to hear that they need to act as if they were already at the next level in order to get a promotion. This is a very good place to apply acting "as if." The coach helped Vanessa explore ways to practice acting "as if" she were already at the next level, along with ways she could advocate for herself.

When asked how her performance shifted in her conversation with her boss, Vanessa responded in a way that showed both greater confidence and thoughtful use of her physicality:

When I get excited, I raise my voice and sit forward. Physically. I wanted his attention. He was deflecting. He would go down a different path with it. I brought the conversation back to me. My body language was not casual at all. Sitting straight up. Leaning forward over his desk. Make sure I had eye contact. Make him as uncomfortable as possible. Let him know I was playing a different role.

For Vanessa, improvisation built an ability to take risks. She also played other roles that helped her grow from a quiet member of the cohort to a very vocal representative of the group. After her manager delayed a response, another leader saw the changes she had made in her leadership and personal styles and created a role for her that involved a promotion. Asked to reflect on the different roles she played during the group meetings, she replied,

The "old Vanessa" was sure and steady. Vanessa in the workshop was zesty, like the Energizer Bunny. The Vanessa who got the new job was persistent. I wasn't going to take "no" lying down. I'm a matured persona now. With the new job, I'm in a new discovery mode: one that is inquisitive yet structured.

Some of the success of the intervention in this case comes from the group work because Vanessa observed the performance of other participants and then chose to modify her own performance based on her observations.

Discussion of the Three Cases

The clients described in this chapter benefited from acting "as if" for different reasons. (Table 13–3 summarizes the three cases for quick reference.) This intervention was an obvious choice for Eric because he was working on an actual presentation. Nathan needed a tool to shift his focus away from his stammer when he spoke to his team and to build his confidence. Vanessa demonstrated that she enjoyed improvisation, so it was logical to suggest the acting "as if" intervention. Not all clients, however, are initially open to this approach. It takes a bit of bravery on the part of the coach or clinician to suggest the approach, some social intelligence to see if there is a true barrier to trying the technique with a client, and some perspective based on professional experience to tailor the strategy to the client's personality, priorities, and situation.

A common question is how to motivate clients to accept an intervention that brings up performance anxiety. One approach is to articulate reasons that will help clients see how the intervention is likely to move them closer to valued goals. Because Eric's promotion was on the line based on the outcome of his performance at the board meeting, he was very motivated to try something new; however, he was initially uncomfortable with some of the roles the coach suggested. The coach needed to have a number of options in order to find the ones that worked. Another approach is to find ways in which the client might already be doing something similar. For example, Nathan was familiar with role-playing while reading aloud to his young children, so the approach did not feel entirely foreign to him, and Vanessa had been involved in improvisation in the leadership development class. Even if there is no known similar behavior, the coach can establish an atmosphere of trust so that clients feel safe enough to experiment without worrying about feeling silly. It can also be helpful to remind them that we all have the experience of being children engaged in pretend play.

The acting "as if" technique can be introduced in a number of ways. For all three clients, this intervention was introduced around session 4 or 5 out of 12 sessions, after the establishment of rapport and trust between the coach and the client. In work with Eric, the coach also explored some of the client's limiting beliefs regarding presentations. Nathan and Vanessa tried some improvisation first to build confidence and competence in the technique. They were then able to act "as if" in broader ways.

Each of the three clients needed to persevere past the initial awkwardness in the first few moments of the session before discovering whether the technique would work for him or her. Evidence that it was working for Eric was that he became more animated and his presentation started to flow. At the conclusion of the session, he told the coach which of the roles felt most comfortable and announced that he was going to rehearse using that role.

TABLE 13–3. Summary of the three case histories

Coaching mode (client name)	Special circumstances	Outcomes
One-on-one coaching (Eric)	Client chose to act as if truly interested (a general quality) rather than emulate a paragon. Extensive practice.	Greater confidence speaking in interorganizational meetings.
Group coaching (Nathan)	Client revealed struggle with stammer. Worked on willingness to be vulnerable with others.	Increased ability to speak in crucial meetings without stammering. Used strengths intentionally to let some people go with grace and soothe fears of others.
Leadership program with one-on-one coaching (Vanessa)	Acting "as if" combined with improvisation in group setting. Worked on self-advocacy in one-on-one sessions.	Increased ability to take risks. Enhanced zest and persistence. Advocated for promotion.

Nathan took a risk in the first group coaching session, which was a win for him and the group, but it was when he presented back to the group and did not stammer that he knew that the role-playing had built his competence. Vanessa knew the approach worked when she took on a leadership role in the final group session and saw the look of shock around the room as she transformed from wallflower to a magnetic master of ceremonies. Each of the three clients had to leap into performing in his or her own zone of proximal development. It was not a linear progression for any of them. This strategy can involve a big jump into trying something new, but because we all acted "as if" when children, perhaps there is "muscle memory."

There are limitations to this technique. Not all clients will be open to this approach. Some might find it seemingly childish or unprofessional. In addition, there is no guarantee that all clients will achieve their desired outcomes from this technique alone. Not all of the personas or characters the coach tried with Eric worked initially. He did not warm up to acting as if he were either Martin Luther King, Jr., or the Baptist preacher, but he persisted until he found what worked for him. Nathan did not speak out at every meeting after learning how to act "as if," because he is more confident with people who know he has a stammer; however, he recently spoke on a panel to a group of 190 people without blocking or becoming nervous. Vanessa did not win over her boss with this technique, but another superior noticed the shift in her performance at work and created a new role for her.

Acting "as if" is a way to get people to see themselves differently. Their mindsets may change from "I can't," "It isn't possible," or "I'm stuck"; to "I can try" or "I can experiment"; and then to "I made it happen." Even for very shy clients who are wary of acting "as if" in the coaching sessions, establishing a clear picture of desired qualities is helpful. These clients can often benefit from reading aloud passages either in the coaching session or at home. Relieved of the responsibility of thinking up what to say, they can focus on expressing the quality with tone, posture, and body movement. For less shy clients, acting "as if" can be presented as a way to experiment with new identities without having to fully commit themselves until they see the outcome. Trying on new behaviors can indirectly change the way they see themselves.

Nathan sums up acting "as if" in this way:

> Think of the first time a kid rides a bike: you're there with them so that they know they are safe, but you let the bike go and they don't realize that they are still fine. Trying on new behaviors in the work context is the same thing. You have the support, the safety net. The next time you do it, it's not as bad as it was the first. You might fall off, but you can get back up again because you have done it and you know you can do it.

Indeed, learning to act "as if" is very much like learning to ride a bike. By being supportive, normalizing the feelings of anxiety or inauthenticity, and finally reflecting back specific positive changes, the coach or clinician provides the training wheels for the first few times a client ventures forth. Then clients can go home and try acting "as if" by themselves as practice before they act "as if" in that next important meeting. Then they will be able to ride toward their destination on their own "as if" they knew how all along.

TAKE-HOME POINTS

- Coaching is a nonclinical intervention focused on improving individuals' behavior, function, and experience but can be focused on strengths as well.

- The coaching strategy of acting "as if" helps individuals enhance their self-efficacy, growth mindset, and character strengths.

- Acting "as if" is a way to get people to see themselves differently.

- The basic structure of this coaching intervention involves five components: determining objectives; asking scaling questions; identifying paragons; leveraging imagination; and reflecting on progress.

REFERENCES

Adler A: Social Interest: A Challenge to Mankind. Translated by Linton J, Vaughan R. London, Faber & Faber, 1938

Adler A: The Individual Psychology of Alfred Adler: A Systematic Presentation in Selections From His Writings. Edited by Ansbacher HL, Ansbacher RR. New York, Harper Torchbooks, 1964

Bandura A: Self-efficacy: toward a unifying theory of behavioral change. Psychol Rev 84(2):191–215, 1977 847061

Bem DJ: Self-perception theory, in Advances in Experimental Social Psychology. Edited by Berkowitz L. New York, Academic Press, 1972, pp 1–62

Berg IK, Szabo P: Brief Coaching for Lasting Solutions. New York, WW Norton, 2005

Biswas-Diener R: Practicing Positive Psychology Coaching: Assessment, Activities, and Strategies for Success. Hoboken, NJ, Wiley, 2010

Biswas-Diener R, Dean B: Positive Psychology Coaching: Putting the Science of Happiness to Work for Your Clients. Hoboken, NJ, Wiley, 2007

Brown S, Vaughan C: Play: How It Shapes the Brain, Opens the Imagination, and Invigorates the Soul. New York, Avery, 2009

Carich MS: Variations of the "as if" technique, in Techniques in Adlerian Psychology. Edited by Carlson J, Slavik S. Washington, DC, Accelerated Development, 1997, pp 153–160

Carlson J, Sperry L: Adlerian psychotherapy as a constructivist psychotherapy, in The Handbook of Constructivist Psychotherapy. Edited by Hoyt MF. San Francisco, CA, Jossey-Bass, 1998, pp 68–82

de Shazer S, Dolan Y: More Than Miracle: The State of the Art of Solution-Focused Brief Therapy. New York, Haworth Press, 2007

Dweck C: Mindset: The New Psychology of Success. New York, Ballantine Books, 2007

Iveson C, George E, Ratner H: Brief Coaching: A Solution-Focused Approach. New York, Routledge, 2012

Niemiec RM: Mindfulness and Character Strengths: A Practical Guide to Flourishing. Boston, MA, Hogrefe, 2014

Nikzadeh E, Soudani M: Evaluating the effectiveness of drama therapy by psychodrama method on psychological well-being and false beliefs of addicts: case study: Persian Gulf Addiction Treatment Center in the city of Bushehr. Rev Eur Stud 8(3):148–155, 2016

Oren SL, Binkert J, Clancy AL: Appreciative Coaching: A Positive Process for Change. San Francisco, CA, Jossey-Bass, 2007

Peterson C, Seligman ME: Character Strengths and Virtues: A Handbook and Classification, Vol 1. New York, Oxford University Press, 2004

Polly S, Britton KH: Character Strengths Matter: How to Live a Full Life. Positive Psychology News, 2015

Salit CR: Performance Breakthrough: A Radical Approach to Success at Work. New York, Hachette Books, 2016

Stanislavski C: An Actor Prepares (1936). Translated by Hapgood ER. New York, Routledge, 1989a

Stanislavski C: Building a Character (1936). Translated by Hapgood ER. New York, Routledge, 1989b

Tarragona M: Positive Identities: Narrative Practices and Positive Psychology (Positive Psychology Workbook Series). Positive Acorn, 2013

Terni P: Solution-focus: bringing positive psychology into the conversation. International Journal of Solution-Focused Practices 3(1):8–16, 2015

VIA Institute on Character: VIA Survey of Character Strengths. 2017. Available at: http://www.viacharacter.org/www/Character-Strengths-Survey. Accessed November 21, 2017.

Vygotsky L: Interaction between learning and development, in Readings on the Development of Children, 2nd Edition. Edited by Gauvain M, Cole M. New York, WH Freeman, 1978, pp 34–41

Watts RE, Peluso PR, Lewis TF: Expanding the Acting As If technique: an Adlerian/constructive integration. J Individ Psychol 61(4):380–387, 2005

Wharton Executive Education: Archive: Nano Tools for Leaders. 2017. Available at: http://executiveeducation.wharton.upenn.edu/thought-leadership/wharton-at-work/nano-tools. Accessed November 21, 2017.

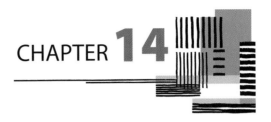

CHAPTER 14

Teaching Positive Psychology in Law School

Daniel S. Bowling III, J.D., M.A.P.P.

Editors' Introduction

This chapter investigates the experience of satisfaction and dissatisfaction in law students and lawyers and describes a highly successful and popular law school course directed at enhancing law student well-being. A detailed description of the course provides a rich picture of how positive interventions are meaningful and effective in an educational setting.

There is considerable evidence, empirical and anecdotal, that the psychological and emotional well-being of U.S. lawyers is not good (Delgado and Stefanic 2008; Patrick 1995; Shiltz 1999). It is thought that their misery begins in law school and continues after graduation, even among those individuals who have obtained postgraduate employment. Some scholars claim that the problems begin even before law school, when pessimists with a risk of depression enter the pressure cooker of law school and get worse as they progress (Seligman et al. 2001).

It would be difficult to design a model of an educational institution that would do a better job of inducing depression and anxiety in a population than does law school (Benjamin et al. 1986). Strict numerical rankings of students who previously dominated undergraduate classrooms, a dearth of cooperative projects, and the systematic stripping of young people's thoughts of idealism and meaning combine to induce helplessness in a population as efficiently as experimental psychologists once did by shocking dogs (Peterson et al. 1976).

There is certainly evidence to support the general hypothesis of the miserable lawyer, both from survey data and empirical research, but I am not alone among scholars in thinking it incomplete and lacking in proper perspective and nuance (Hull 1999). After years of teaching second- and third-year law students at Duke University about the science of well-being and its application in the law, as well as having the students voluntarily experiment with personality testing, I find that nothing has changed my opinion. Of course law students are stressed, with emotional peaks and valleys on an almost weekly basis, and fearful of their job prospects. However, it is my opinion that as a whole they are more normal, well-adjusted, and capable of happiness than academic researchers and popular commentators give them credit for being.

In fact, among the hundreds of students over the years who have voluntarily experimented in my classes with psychological surveys, such as the Values in Action (VIA) Survey of Character Strengths (Peterson and Seligman 2004), results have been generally similar to those of the adult U.S. population (results obtained in private surveying of law firm clients). Although this testing was designed to familiarize students with basic tools for measuring well-being scientifically as well as to analyze the legal implications of personality testing, and was not subject to rigorous testing standards (and was done voluntarily, anonymously, and with no grade or other reward attached), the findings do present an interesting picture—one resistive of conventional wisdom—of a rather large group of second- and third-year students at one law school. I also acknowledge that the experience of a student population at a highly ranked law school, with high employment rates, might differ from that of other student populations.

I do not intend to diminish or trivialize the fact that reported incidents of depression among law students in general are high (Dammeyer and Nunez 1999). However, law students are not the only graduate students with high rates of depression and suicide; there is evidence that students in medical, pharmaceutical, and Ph.D. programs suffer from many of the same maladies. One multi-school study found that 25% of medical students showed symptoms of depression and 6.6% reported suicidal ideation (Goebert et al. 2009).

Few people, however, suggest drastically modifying medical and doctoral studies programs because of these problems. Although it cannot be ignored that the structure and methods of a U.S. law school produce distress among certain students (Benjamin et al. 2008; Krieger 2002), anyone who would use these statistics and stories to significantly change the pedagogical structure of law school and the way associates are trained in large firms would be ignoring the fact that U.S. law schools produce some of the finest lawyers in the world. Furthermore, many if not most lawyers live productive and fulfilled lives (Heinz et al. 1999; Hull 1999). It is also unrealistic to expect that wholesale changes in the law school model will be driven by well-being statistics, so the more pragmatic action would be to focus on ways to ameliorate the most extreme stressors of law school and law practice (Bowling 2015; Brafford 2014).

Law Course on Well-Being and the Practice of Law

The roots of the course titled "Well-Being and the Practice of Law" lie in a chance hallway discussion I had in 2009 with a senior member of the faculty, Professor John Weistart, about the psychological issues facing the profession. As head of the curriculum committee, he suggested I propose a course on the topic outlined below, and the course was approved. It has been offered for the last 6 years, has become one of the highest-rated courses at Duke, and is oversubscribed each year. I attribute this to the subject matter, not the instructor.

Course Description

The introductory paragraph of the syllabus describes the thesis of the course:

> "Well-Being and the Practice of Law" examines why the "pursuit of happiness," a phrase written by a lawyer, has proved futile for many members of the legal profession and those aspiring to its ranks. There is considerable data and anecdotal evidence indicating that lawyers and law students suffer from greater rates of depression and anxiety than other professions, along with accompanying social maladies such as substance abuse and stress-related illness. There is also evidence of high career dissatisfaction among lawyers, and many others are leaving the profession or performing well below their capability. This seems unfathomable given the high levels of education, affluence, and respect lawyers enjoy (or will enjoy), all of which are factors that predict happiness and job satisfaction in other areas of life. Importantly, some research indicates these problems *begin in law school*. This implies that something happens between graduation from college and the beginning of practice that negatively impacts life satisfaction at a rate far beyond other professional or graduate educational models.

Pedagogical Focus and Method

In addition to examining the issues set forth in the introduction to this chapter, the class focuses on very important, but underexplored, questions: What is the impact of lawyers' alleged unhappiness on legal professionalism? Are well-being and professionalism interrelated? Or, in layperson's terms, is a happier lawyer a better, more ethical one? If so, why, and what should legal institutions do to increase lawyer well-being?

The class first examines what *happiness* is—and is not—and how it has been defined through the ages, acknowledging that the term means different things to different people and researchers (Adler 2013). It then reviews the research to date on lawyers and psychological health. Following this theoretical grounding, the class examines the scientific data and academic literature on lawyer maladies, and looks for holes in the collective wisdom (e.g., explore reasons why many lawyers and law students are quite content—happy, even). After acknowledging the very real problems of the profession, the class then grapples with the legitimate question many lawyers and law professors ask: *So what?* Who said lawyers are supposed to be happy?

The class experiments with interventions designed to increase well-being, both to become familiar with tools in the area and to use them for future application or study. In particular, as discussed at more length below (see subsection "Character Strengths"), the class explores psychological traits and character strengths and the importance of aligning them with career choices in law practice and life, and considers what actions one can take to increase one's overall well-being.

Class participation is very important, a point made clear from the outset. Out of respect for the different classroom participation styles of introverts and extroverts, I provide opportunities outside class for credited participation, such as informal papers and online chats. I emphasize participation because the students' views on the issues and questions presented are expressed via engagement in application exercises, and these exercises are important to the progression of the course. Student participation is also important in developing my understanding of law students and what is important in their lives.

Grading Policy

There is no exam in the course. Grades are based largely on a final paper, but weight is also given to participation and involvement with the course. The course is not an "easy A"; it is graded on a strict curve, with the median set by school policy. It was very important, given my belief that well-being should be in the mainstream of the law school curriculum, that the course be graded in the same manner as contract or torts law, rather than by the "softer" pass-fail method. That does not mean I try to conduct class through the brutal Socratic examination famed in law school legend; instead, I look for ways to induce positive emotions throughout each session, believing this to be a far better method to "broaden and build" student minds (Fredrickson 2001).

What I look for in assigning grades is that over the course of the semester, each student forms his or her own theory of well-being that is presented in the student's writing and class participation. The hypothesis need not support the central premise of the class; grades are based on how well the student synthesizes the readings and discussions along with the student's own experience into a cohesive and insightful theory on the relationship of well-being and professionalism. An excellent final paper shows a firm grasp of the material and issues presented, is well organized with appropriate references, is persuasively written, and engages the reader intellectually.

Reflection Papers

The students write a short reflection paper after each class based on the topic presented, the readings, the activities, and their reaction to them. These reflection papers are more like well-crafted blog posts than formal academic papers and are approximately one page in length. These papers are not formally graded but do count toward the 15-page writing requirement for a one-credit course under American Bar Association accreditation standards.

Reading Assignments

There is no textbook or casebook. Reading assignments, selected from the academic literature on lawyer well-being as well as positive psychology, are posted online.

Final Writing Requirement

The bulk of each student's grade is based on a formal paper due at the end of the semester. I give the students leeway in style and topic, but many students—unaccustomed to writing theoretical academic essays—struggle to get started. Therefore, I provide the following prompts:

1. Why is happiness in the law so elusive for so many according to survey data?
2. Is it possible for professionalism and the highest ethical behavior to flourish when lawyers show high rates of mental distress? If not, should legal institutions encourage well-being?
3. What roles do personality, emotions, and character strengths play in the lives of lawyers? Should firms and lawyers take personality into account in career choices, assignments, and so forth?
4. What does scientific research into "happiness" have to offer the legal profession, and how can you apply it in your own life and career?
5. How can lawyer well-being be advocated in a persuasive manner to leaders of legal institutions? What actions would you encourage law schools and firms to take?

In the Classroom

The class counts for one academic credit. It meets six times during the semester, for a little over 2 hours per class (13 hours' face-to-face time per credit is required by the American Bar Association). It is intense, with considerable discussion, debate, and more than a little laughter. Through trial and error, I have learned what is important to the students and what is not. I have also tried not to induce depression by the (necessary) focus on the evidentiary basis of lawyer maladaptation, so striking the right balance between *description* of the evidence and *prescription* for improving one's well-being is a challenge each year. Out of the many things I have covered over the last 6 years, the three most important, necessary, and effective are set out below.

Philosophical Grounding

At the outset, I introduce theories and questions about the definition of *well-being*, its history, and current research in positive psychology. The class spends considerable time focusing on definitions of *happiness* and *well-being*, in particular, distinguishing scholarly approaches from more popular notions. Specifically, I concentrate on Aristotelian theories of well-being, or *eudaimonia*, which are well suited to lawyers and law students (Graham 1995–96).

Aristotle believed that a purpose of life is to seek well-being, which for the purposes of teaching law students can best be understood as relating to character strengths and virtues and their employment in the civic good (Bowling 2015). More useful for the purposes of the class is the Aristotelian notion of *intrinsic motivation*—wanting to do something because one wants it for itself, not for what it represents.

It is not difficult for students to understand the links between intrinsic motivation—wanting to be a lawyer for its own sake—and extrinsic motivations—such as money or, more simply, something to do with one's life after obtaining a liberal arts degree—for attending law school. From there, the connection with true happiness in the practice of law becomes clearer (Bowling 2015).

As the semester advances, more sophisticated links between legal ethics and *eudaimonia* are developed by and for the students. Aristotle, in his *Ethics*, argues that true well-being arises from the pursuit of virtue (Melchert 2002). For lawyers, this entails two components: 1) the use of one's legal skills to the best of one's ability, or, in other words, the seeking of "excellence"; and 2) the pursuit of an intrinsically moral goal, a purpose or a cause that is of personal importance.

At the end of the semester, the students write short "meaning" papers, in which they imagine a look back at their life and career and reflect on what was important and what was not. Invariably, the students' reflections are well informed by the Aristotelian principles taught at the outset.

Character Strengths

The most effective and sustainable application exercise involves the measurement and exploration of character strengths. Although *character* can be defined in different ways, I focus in the class on positive dispositions using the VIA Survey of Character Strengths (available for no cost at http://authentic happiness.com). This measure was created in part by Christopher Peterson and Martin Seligman to measure 24 positive characteristics (or strengths), such as authenticity, bravery, creativity, curiosity, and fairness. These characteristics were chosen according to several criteria, including that they were seen as relatively universal, fulfilling to the individual, morally valued by individuals and societies, trait-like, measureable, and distinctive (Peterson and Seligman 2004).

Numerous studies have been conducted on character strengths, and the results suggest that strengths in general are linked to better physical, mental, social, and occupational outcomes. For individual law students, using one's top-ranked strength relates to lower likelihoods of depression and stress and increased life satisfaction (Peterson and Peterson 2009). Similarly, a growing number of studies suggest that using top strengths daily relates to higher well-being in work and life (Rath and Harter 2010).

Somewhat surprisingly, character strengths overall, including strengths identified by the study as related to "love of learning," are negatively correlated with grades in law school (albeit slightly), according to a study conducted several years ago at two selective law schools (Kern and Bowling 2015). However, that study did not measure outcomes beyond grades, and in our class at Duke, the students review studies showing character strengths in law practice align with career satisfaction and success in a way that is consistent with the results from other business and professional domains (Snyder et al. 2015).

Students who are interested in their own results voluntarily take the VIA survey online and report their results in class. Although this study is not scientifically rigorous and not designed for research purposes, the results over the years have been remarkably consistent. Law students score very high in the intellectual strengths such as critical thinking, not surprisingly, but also high in more emotional strengths such as capacity to love. Perhaps, students suggest, the popular image of the heartless lawyer is an inaccurate one.

A favorite in-class exercise is for students to imagine and design a law firm in which different practice areas are populated with persons of strengths appropriate to that area. Human resources law, for example, might attract lawyers high in social intelligence; corporate transactional law might call for students high in diligence; firm management might call for leadership strengths; and so on. The exercise is a fun one for the class and prompts reflection in the students as to the importance of strengths alignment in careers. Numerous students have reported that learning about their strengths helped them shape career choices in a positive manner.

Resilience Exercises

Over the years, I have experimented by having students do different hands-on exercises that would be familiar to anyone exposed to the positive psychology literature: writing gratitude letters, focusing on "three good things" in one's life, meditation, and so on (Seligman 2004). Occasionally, I have invited guest experts to conduct the exercises, but over time I have relied less and less on outside speakers; it is difficult for the students to become comfortable with an outsider during a single class, so I do my best to conduct the training event alone.

Some exercises have not gone well (e.g., my inexpert attempt to conduct a meditation session). Others have been fun but trifling in their effects. Based on my observations in and after class, and from anecdotal evidence as to what "works" in a student's life, exercises that form the basis of the U.S. Army's resilience training efforts, discussed below, have been the most effective.

The exercises, grounded for the most part in the cognitive-behavioral literature, are credible to the students in part because they are framed in the context of the military. Perhaps this is because some lawyers love war metaphors: they are constantly "doing battle" or "donning armor" for trial. Metaphorical flourishes aside, there are parallels between the life of a lawyer and that of a soldier in that both professions involve constant stress and failure is not an option. It is hard for students to dismiss positive psychology as "too soft" when soldiers practice it.

The army resilience training program started in 2009 when then–chief of staff General William Casey ordered his staff to develop training to respond to increased incidents of suicide and posttraumatic stress disorder among troops facing repeated deployment. They chose psychologists from the University of Pennsylvania to develop a program to teach positive psychology skills to the 1.1 million men and women in uniform. Using culturally normative terms such as *mental toughness* and *battle-mind*, the program is grounded in the resilience literature and teaches techniques to reduce pessimism and anxiety—the building blocks of stress disorders. The training also addresses emotional awareness, something not usually discussed or developed during basic training, one would imagine (Reivich et al. 2011).

Two exercises from the army's resilience tool kit have become a staple of my class. Many readers will be familiar with the techniques, so I describe them here in only the broadest terms.

ACTIVE CONSTRUCTIVE RESPONDING

Research shows that relationships between individuals can be improved when one responds in a certain way to the *good* news of another (Gable et al. 2004). Humans have little trouble in responding appropriately, if inarticulately, to news of another's tragedy or hardship. Few laugh in another's face when told of the death of a loved one. However, people are not particularly good at responding to the good news of another. They might point out the potential problems if a scenario is presented as good or, worse, ignore it altogether or change the subject.

This tendency is exacerbated in competitive environments like law school. It is hard for a student without a job to respond excitedly to a friend announcing a six-figure offer. However, the recipient of the news must respond actively, and affirmatively, if he or she is to strengthen emotional bonds with the friend.

This constructive responding exercise is not difficult to do in class. The students break into pairs and then practice sharing news and responding. The challenge is for each student to find his or her own authentic voice so it does not sound faked, which is not easy at first. For weeks after the classroom exercise, I see students practicing on one another in the hallways. The exercise works.

CHALLENGING NEGATIVE THOUGHTS

Each person has an internal voice, or narrator, interpreting events in his or her life. Often, particularly in individuals under stress such as law students, the narrator is dark and pessimistic, warning of threats and dangers and creating cascading emotional responses whether those dangers are real or not. Although this is an evolutionarily adaptive trait in humans, in the modern world it can create unnecessary anxiety.

To introduce students to techniques to challenge their negative thoughts, I use the ABC model familiar to cognitive therapists as modified for army training (Reivich et al. 2011). The idea is to teach students to identify a potentially stressful event (A, for activating), consider their thoughts about the event (B, for beliefs), and trace the emotional consequences (C, for consequences). The students will be given a hypothetical activating event (e.g., "Your professor won't make eye contact with you"), identify their instinctive beliefs about the event ("She hates me"), and assess the consequences (e.g., sadness, anxiety). Through repeated exercises such as this (considering different reasons for the activating event, such as the professor may have been distracted by an overdue research project), the students learn to start challenging negative beliefs about activating events (if no evidence exists of their negativity) and thereby moderate the emotional consequences.

Although the model is a bit cumbersome for the classroom without trained facilitators roaming the room, the students adapt to the methodology after I reframe it as "cross-examining" negative thoughts. In other words, law students can use the skepticism and demand for evidentiary proof ingrained in them in other classes to strengthen their cognitive muscles.

LAW STUDENT VOICES

In this chapter, I have offered my impressions of what law students are thinking. My impressions are taken from classroom conversations, student papers, and individual meetings and conversations. The students are a cross-section of Duke University law students, and I believe they are a representative sample of law students at a selective school. I have read hundreds of their papers during the last several years and spent countless hours in and out of class with the students, and through these interactions I have been provided a privileged look into the inner life of those on the cusp of entering the practice of law. Out of respect for their privacy, I do not name any student or include anything directly from students' writings (although I maintain all writings on file). I am confident, however, that my impressions are accurate.

It should also be noted that although the students do not represent a scientific sample (was there selection bias among the students who chose this elective?), they represent a statistically significant group, approximately 10% of the second- and third-year classes. As such, I have casually observed what seems to be a wide distribution of personalities and attitudes, from an almost Panglossian optimism and cheerfulness in some, to a gloominess that a clinician might diagnose as evidence of serious depression in others.

I have tried to present as balanced a sample of student impressions as I can, including those at the extremes, from students who think this entire issue is irrelevant nonsense, to those who think law schools should be torn down because of the harm they inflict on young people, to those who think the course is the most important one they ever took. Generally, however, these extremes are rare, and common themes have emerged over the years.

As to the central thesis of the course, the students wrestle with the notion that well-being is synonymous with being an effective representative of a client and member of a profession, perhaps because the notion is quite foreign to them. Many seem surprised when I share the results of an unpublished survey I conducted in 2010 at a large Atlanta-based law firm, where 77% of the attorneys who took the survey ($N=107$) agreed with the proposition linking well-being and professionalism (data on file with the author).

Some students agree with certain scholars (e.g., Kronman 1999) that well-being and legal professionalism are inseparable; employers and law schools have a heretofore unrecognized ethical duty to ensure well-being among students and employees. Others, perhaps a majority of the students, see this view as a little extreme. Although they may recognize the importance of promoting well-being, viewing it as an ethical duty might go too far and raise too many issues. These individuals might ask, "How would this duty be enforced? What measurement tools would be used? How would we deal with external factors causing unhappiness?"

A general consensus has formed among students over the years: although employers might not have a duty to ensure their workers' well-being, employers do have good and logical reasons to promote their workers' well-being. The practice of law will always involve unpleasant or tedious tasks, but as my students who have joined a law review will attest, even the worst job can be made better by working together with others.

The most consistent theme among the students is that well-being among law students should be taken seriously by law schools, from an informational standpoint and/or by addressing it through formal curricula such as this course. Virtually no students, other than the few holding the extreme views mentioned above, claim that the well-being of fellow classmates during law school is meaningless.

Another theme, present to a varying extent in different years depending on the job market, is the impact of postgraduate employment on student well-being. Surprisingly, those with job offers from the biggest and most competitive of law firms do not describe or present themselves as significantly "happier" than those with offers from less prestigious firms or institutions, or even those with no offers at all. Indeed, one study showed that law students with higher Law School Admission Test (LSAT) scores reported lower life satisfaction in law school. This is interesting because there is a correlation among high LSAT scores and law school grades, and employment with large law firms after law school (Gottfredson et al. 2008).

My theory on this seeming anomaly, based on student papers, is that the reason individuals chose to go to law school greatly colors their perceptions of the law school experience. Those students who went to law school "to become a lawyer"—that is, those intrinsically drawn to the study of law—seem less troubled by their after-school job status. Those students extrinsically motivated by the financial rewards of big-firm practice seem to have more trouble enjoying the journey to get there; or, alternatively, perhaps they are worried about their future because much of the anecdotal and survey data on lawyer misery comes from the experiences of associates at big firms (Shiltz 1999).

CONCLUSION

Cynics might claim that law students are defined more by their generation than by the fact that they are law students. According to popular wisdom, millennials tend to be whiny, self-absorbed, focused on their own well-being and state in life, and disrespectful of institutions and adults. As law students, such millennials are apt to be smart, articulate, and persuasive writers. Thus, the cynics would argue that there is an inordinate focus on the problems with law students and young lawyers because these individuals are more prone than other young people to talk and blog about their state.

There are two problems with this claim by critics in my opinion. First, the evidence of lawyer and law student distress is decades old and cross-generational, as a review of the references herein quickly shows (Benjamin et al. 1990). Second, I don't believe the claim. The students I know are decent, likable, hard-working, and sincere people, and probably not much different from other graduate students for whom pressure and uncertainty are constantly present in their lives.

I strongly believe a course similar to "Well-Being and the Practice of Law" is applicable in other disciplines, particularly medicine. I have tried to be specific in this chapter about its design and implementation in the hope that others will be inspired to create and teach similar courses, not only in law school but also in other professional graduate schools. These types of courses are needed.

TAKE-HOME POINTS

- Well-being is an essential element of being an effective professional.

- Professionals can effectively enhance their well-being through the application of positive psychology techniques.

- There is strong demand for positive psychology in postgraduate education.

- Positive psychology theory and techniques can be taught effectively in professional schools.

References

Adler MD: Happiness surveys and public policy: what's the use? Duke Law Journal 62:1509–1601, 2013

Benjamin GA, Kazniak A, Sales B, et al: The role of legal education in producing psychological distress among law students and lawyers. Law Soc Inq 37:225–252, 1986

Benjamin GA, Darling EJ, Sales B: The prevalence of depression, alcohol abuse, and cocaine abuse among United States lawyers. Int J Law Psychiatry 13(3):233–246, 1990 2228368

Bowling DS: Lawyers and their elusive pursuit of happiness: does it matter? Duke Forum for Law and Social Change 7:37–52, 2015

Brafford AM: Building the positive law firm: the legal profession at its best (master's capstone). August 1, 2014. Available at: http://repository.upenn.edu/cgi/viewcontent.cgi?article=1063&context=mapp_capstone. Accessed November 21, 2017.

Dammeyer MM, Nunez N: Anxiety and depression among law students: current knowledge and future directions. Law Hum Behav 23(1):55–73, 1999 10100457

Delgado R, Stefanic J: Can lawyers find happiness? Syracuse Law Rev 58:261–275, 2008

Flores M, Arce RM: Why are lawyers killing themselves? CNN, January 20, 2014. Available at: http://www.cnn.com/2014/01/19/us/lawyer-suicides/. Accessed November 21, 2017.

Fredrickson BL: The role of positive emotions in positive psychology: the broaden-and-build theory of positive emotions. Am Psychol 56(3):218–226, 2001 11315248

Gable SL, Reis HT, Impett EA, et al: What do you do when things go right? The intrapersonal and interpersonal benefits of sharing positive events. J Pers Soc Psychol 87(2):228–245, 2004 15301629

Goebert D, Thompson D, Takeshita J, et al: Depressive symptoms in medical students and residents: a multischool study. Acad Med 84(2):236–241, 2009 19174678

Gottfredson NC, Panter AT, Daye CE, et al: Identifying predictors of law student life satisfaction. J Legal Educ 58(4):520–530, 2008

Graham LM: Aristotle's ethics and the virtuous lawyer: part one of a study on legal ethics and clinical education. Journal of the Legal Profession 20:5–49, 1995–96

Heinz J, Hull K, Harter AA: Lawyers and their discontents: findings from a survey of the Chicago bar. Indiana Law J 74(3):735–758, 1999

Hull K: Cross-examining the myth of lawyers' misery. Vanderbilt Law Rev 52:971–972, 1999

Kern ML, Bowling DS: Character strengths and academic performance in law students. J Res Pers 55:25–29, 2015

Krieger LS: Psychological insights: why our students and graduates suffer, and what we might do about it. Journal of the Association of Legal Writing Directors, 2002. Available at: http://papers.ssrn.com/sol3/papers.cfm?abstract_id=1095636. Accessed November 21, 2017.

Kronman A: Legal professionalism. Fla State Univ Law Rev 27:3–4, 1999

Melchert N: Aristotle: the reality of the world: the good life, in The Great Conversation: A Historical Introduction to Philosophy, 4th Edition. Boston, MA, McGraw-Hill, 2002, pp 186–198

Dolan M: Miserable with the legal life. More and more lawyers hate their jobs , surveys find. Commercial pressure, burnout, and a glut of rivals are blamed. Los Angeles Times, June 27, 1995. Available at: http://articles.latimes.com/1995-06-27/news/mn-17704_1_legal-life. Accessed November 21, 2017.

Peterson C, Seligman ME: Character Strengths and Virtues: A Handbook and Classification, Vol 1. New York, Oxford University Press, 2004

Peterson C, Maier SF, Seligman ME: Learned helplessness: theory and evidence. J Exp Psychol Gen 105:3–46, 1976

Peterson TD, Peterson EW: Stemming the tide of law student depression: what law schools need to learn from the science of positive psychology. Yale J Health Policy Law Ethics 9(2):357–434, 2009 19725388

Rath T, Harter J: Well Being: The Five Essential Elements. New York, Gallup Press, 2010

Reivich KJ, Seligman ME, McBride S: Master resilience training in the U.S. Army. Am Psychol 66(1):25–34, 2011 21219045

Seligman ME: Authentic Happiness: Using the New Positive Psychology to Realize Your Potential for Lasting Fulfillment. New York, Simon & Schuster, 2004

Seligman ME, Verkuil PR, Kang TH: Why lawyers are unhappy. Cardozo Law Rev 23:33–53, 2001

Shiltz P: On being a happy, healthy, and ethical member of an unhappy, unhealthy, and unethical profession. Vanderbilt Law Rev 52:871–951, 1999

Snyder P: Super women lawyers: a study of character strengths. Arizona Summit Law Rev 8(3):261-316, 2015

Index

*Page numbers printed in **boldface** type refer to tables and figures.*